LOSE
WEIGHT
HERE

LOSE WEIGHT HERE

THE METABOLIC SECRET TO TARGET STUBBORN FAT AND FIX YOUR PROBLEM AREAS

DR. JADE TETA, ND, and DR. KEONI TETA, ND
FOUNDERS OF METABOLIC EFFECT

RODALE.

RODALE *wellness*

Live happy. Be healthy. Get inspired.

Sign up today to get exclusive access to our authors, exclusive bonuses,
and the most authoritative, useful, and cutting-edge information on health,
wellness, fitness, and living your life to the fullest.

Visit us online at RodaleWellness.com
Join us at RodaleWellness.com/Join

© 2015 by Jade Teta, ND, CSCS, and Keoni Teta, ND, LAc, CSCS

Trade hardcover first published by Rodale Inc. in April 2015.
Trade paperback first published by Rodale Inc. in June 2016.

Rodale books may be purchased for business or promotional use or for special sales.
For information, please write to:
Special Markets Department, Rodale Inc., 733 Third Avenue, New York, NY 10017

Printed in the United States of America
Rodale Inc. makes every effort to use acid-free ∞, recycled paper ♲.

Graphic on page 198 courtesy of Epel, McEwen, Seeman, Matthews, Castellazzo, et al.
"Stress and Body Shape: Stress-Induced Cortisol Secretion Is Consistently Greater Among Women with Central Fat." *Psychosomatic Medicine* 62 (2000): 623–32.
Breakfast Casserole (page 109) courtesy of Emily Saunders and
Coconut Baked Oatmeal (page 110) courtesy of Jillian Teta
Illustrations on pages 36, 49, 61, 87, 96, 122 & 194 by John Stevens
Exercise photographs by Lisa Brewer
Candid photographs submitted by success story participants
Book design by Christina Gaugler

Library of Congress Cataloging-in-Publication Data is on file with the publisher.
ISBN 978–1–62336–476–2 hardcover
ISBN 978–1–62336–785–5 paperback

Distributed to the trade by Macmillan

4 6 8 10 9 7 5 3   paperback

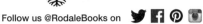

Follow us @RodaleBooks on

We inspire and enable people to improve their lives and the world around them.

This book is dedicated to the dream that one day individualized medicine will take the place of one-size-fits-all protocols and that doctors will invest in teaching their patients how to fully understand and honor their own metabolic uniqueness.

Contents

Introduction

We both can remember one of the first personal training clients we ever had pointing to the back of her arm and saying, "How do I lose weight *right here*?" Now, years later in our clinic, we are confronted with the same question again and again—men distraught over stubborn chest fat they call "man boobs," women complaining about saddlebags and inner thigh fat, and both men and women asking us to help them get rid of belly fat that stays no matter what they do.

But you know better than that, don't you? You know you can't lose weight where you want to. It simply does not work that way. You're born to be a certain shape—be it a pear, or an apple, or a ruler—and you're destined to remain that way for life. At least that is what the diet books, workout gurus, and health bloggers have told you.

After all, anyone who has ever exhaustively exercised and religiously dieted in an attempt to reshape his or her body can tell you that, in many ways, it is an exercise in futility. Can you relate? Sure, you go on a diet and you lose weight and tone up, but despite your best efforts, you are disappointed when your large pear shape merely becomes a smaller, and usually mushier, pear shape. If your thighs, belly, hips, and butt were problem areas before the diet, they'll usually remain problems even after you drastically cut calories and slog away on the treadmill. Muscle-building exercises like weight lifting often backfire and give you a puffy, waterlogged look. Even worse, the best results never last: Diets are notorious for their fleeting results, and most people will regain all of their lost weight—or worse, end up even fatter than they were *before* they started dieting.

And where does the weight always seem to grow back fastest? In the stubborn problem areas people are most determined to target, such as the belly, butt, hips, and thighs.

Why does this happen? Your metabolism does not work like a calculator the way the calorie zealots and diet pushers want you to believe. It does not work like a chemistry set either, the way the low-carb fanatics and insulin junkies want you to believe. In reality, there is no exact magic mathematical formula or hormonal-chemistry mixture that leads to sustained and lasting fat loss for all. In fact, both of these approaches will just as easily create the metabolic damage described above.

But there's good news: You can escape the diet trap, fix your metabolism for good, and change the shape of your body—really. When you fully embrace the concepts we outline in this book, you likely will never view diet, weight loss, and metabolism the same way again. The metabolic secret we outline is the key to losing weight, keeping it off for good, and losing fat right where you want to.

We're Jade and Keoni Teta, both of us doctors of naturopathic medicine. As integrative physicians and weight-loss specialists, we specialize in correcting metabolic disturbances that lead to weight gain and physiological dysfunction, and we've been perfecting the Lose Weight Here plan since 2004, when we launched Metabolic Effect as a boot camp shortly after returning home from medical school. Since then, we've expanded our practice, growing our metabolic clinic into a virtual health resource that consults with thousands of international clients each year. We wrote a best-selling diet book called *The Metabolic Effect Diet* and built a physical and online training center that has now certified thousands of professionals to teach our metabolic methodology. In the process, we developed a unique clinical practice that marries our specialties of natural medicine, strength training and conditioning, and hormonal approaches to weight loss. We've collected all of our know-how and put it into these pages, and with this plan we are going to reprogram the way you think and teach you to revise your traditional weight-management techniques by identifying and optimizing the two components that are essential for successful weight loss: low calories and hormonal balance.

A NEW APPROACH

Simply put, dieting is making you fat, and it has made your metabolism defective. That defect is not only keeping you from losing weight, but also slowly making you fatter and your stubborn fatty areas even more stubborn. Up until this moment, you have been operating under the assumption that your metabolism is mapped out like this:

Calorie Reduction = Weight Loss = Balanced Metabolism

In reality, weight loss and your metabolism work more like this:

Balanced Metabolism = Natural Calorie Reduction = Permanent Weight Loss

As we said, two things are required to lose weight: low calories and hormonal balance. The popular "eat less, exercise more" approach (which most diet books and programs push in one way or another) easily lowers calories, but also disrupts hormonal physiology. As a consequence, key metabolic hormones like leptin, insulin, thyroid, and others shift in a way that causes increased hunger, unpredictable energy levels, relentless cravings, and a dramatically slowed metabolic rate. All of these changes mean any short-term weight-loss results you enjoyed quickly turn into long-term metabolic damage. Eventually, you will regain the weight you lost, more of that weight will end up in the hard-to-lose fat areas you were trying to get rid of in the first place, and it will be even more stubborn the next time you diet. In other words, if you want to get fatter and make your fat more stubborn, dieting is the best way to accomplish it.

The Lose Weight Here program is something entirely different from what you've experienced before—and it's far more effective. It teaches you how you can reverse metabolic damage and weight-loss resistance to see weight-loss and body-shaping results fast. To get lean and change the shape of your body quickly, you've got to stop counting calories and endlessly working out. Approaching things in this new way works with the natural "thermostat" nature of the body, decreasing the potential for metabolic compensation and weight regain. It also adjusts the biochemistry of stubborn fat areas so they are more likely to burn fat at rates similar to the rest of the body. In other words: You can stop uneven fat loss and lose fat exactly where you want to lose it.

As we did in our first book, we want to show you how to make your metabolism work for you. In *The Metabolic Effect Diet*, we demonstrated the difference between weight loss from cutting calories and fat loss from balancing metabolic hormones. By triggering the body's hormones to burn fat, not muscle, you can lose fat at an astounding rate. The Lose Weight Here plan takes the fat-loss concept one step further, showing you how to speed fat loss from specific areas to achieve real shape change. We will get your hunger, energy, and cravings—which we'll refer to collectively as your HEC (pronounced *heck*)—in check, and get you on the road to becoming the you you've always wanted to be. And this time, you will have the tools to maintain it for life.

IS SPOT REDUCTION REALLY POSSIBLE?

First, to be clear, this book is *not* about spot reduction. Actual spot reduction, the way you might be imagining it—exercising one spot with the hope of shrinking it—is not possible from a practical standpoint. You cannot exercise a particular area and burn significant amounts of fat from that area alone. The body burns fat from all over. It is just that in certain areas, fat burns at a much slower rate than in others. What you will be learning in this book is how to take the brakes off *stubborn* fat so it burns at the same rate as fat elsewhere in your body. That *is* possible, but dieting and doing targeted exercises is exactly the wrong way to go about it. In this book, we will teach you how it really works. That means a diet, exercise, rest, relaxation, and metabolic overhaul is in order to start the process and get rid of the trouble spots for good.

REVERSING THE DAMAGE

The good news is that you can reverse the metabolic damage you've sustained and land the body you've always dreamed of having by combining hormonal fat-burning science, our method of metabolic training, and our clinical, practical work developed by helping tens of thousands of people achieve their goals as patients in our clinic, members of our online community, or readers of our book. We'll give you the basics—what you should eat, how you should exercise, and how to get your best rest during the three different stages of your journey. We will arm you to be diet detectives by teaching you how to assess, investigate, and modify (or AIM, as we call it) our advice to work for you, because, of course, one size does not fit all. We are going to explain three basic keys to you first: metabolic damage and the Law of Metabolic Compensation, the Law of Metabolic Multitasking, and the Law of Metabolic Individuality, which will show you the way to create your personalized weight-loss program for targeted fat loss and body reshaping. These laws are the keys to changing your body shape and avoiding the trap that swallows up two-thirds of all dieters and makes them fatter than they were before they started dieting.

After that, we'll take you through the three stages of our program to get your body where you want it to be. There are two ways to create the calorie deficit you need for fat loss while balancing the metabolic hormones in a way that ensures that the fat stays off. We'll start you off with the Eat Less, Exercise Less (or ELEL) phase, which to some of you might seem counterintuitive. Then we have you enter the Eat More, Exercise More (or EMEM) phase. Those two protocols form the core of our approach, and while they might require an adjustment in your thinking, they are the most powerful fat-burning protocols we have ever seen. These first steps will help to attack stubborn fat by breaking the dieting cycle for good and healing your metabolism. We'll share some success stories along the way.

We will also be giving you a new goal: no goal. Well, not exactly. But you will need to let go of your obsession with numbers and instead focus on your body shape. At its core, this book is about producing a body shape that truly reflects the effort you put into your diet, exercise, and lifestyle. We'll help women achieve the coveted hourglass figure (the healthiest shape for women, defined as symmetrical waist-to-chest and waist-to-hip ratios) and help men carve the sought-after V shape (the healthiest shape for men).

We have a shape calculator online at metaboliceffect.com/me-shape-calculator that will help you understand how your shape is changing and whether you are achieving an appropriate ratio of muscle to fat. Rather than pounds and inches, your guide will be the way you feel and look in pictures, and the measurable reshaping of your body.

IT'S TIME FOR A TURNAROUND

It's time to banish the saddlebags and trouble spots from your body and take control—without going hungry, without overexercising, and without depriving yourself of the fuel you need to stay healthy. The solution: the Lose Weight Here plan. The pages of this book will change your life—forever. Based on our experience with our clients, you will likely see results in as little as 2 weeks. But the best part is, the results won't stop there. Using our unique approach, you'll keep losing weight and reshaping yourself until you hit your ideal weight and shape. Say good-bye to the stubborn trouble spots that have plagued you at every weight. It's time to reshape your body for good.

The plan in this book is logical and simple, with head-turning results that start to occur within a very short time frame. It's evidence based, will achieve rapid results, and has been proven to reshape your body and your stubborn spots. Most importantly, it gives you the tools to personalize the program to make it effective and appropriate just for you.

Let's go get it.

For more resources, information, and support:

Follow us on Twitter @metaboliceffect, @jadeteta, @keoniteta, and on Facebook.com/metaboliceffect.

Check out our blog or consider joining one of our online programs at metaboliceffect.com.

Tune in to the Metabolic Effect Podcast on iTunes.

Part I

The Science
of Targeted
Weight Loss

Andrea

At 48, Andrea went from a "skinny-fat apple shape" to a perimenopausal "fat, apple-pear shape." Her hormones were out of whack, and she was being treated by a physician for a few border-line issues. She was also a diet fad junkie jumping from program to program, but nothing helped. She thought she was stuck in her body because of her age and health issues. The Lose Weight Here plan changed everything for her. Just a few weeks into the program, she'd shed 13 pounds and more than 8 inches

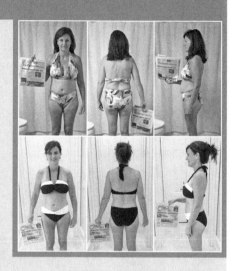

between her hips and waist. Better, she got rid of what she called "bra bulge" and no longer dreamed of getting a breast reduction.

More important, she got used to her metabolism, was able to reduce her stress, and stopped staying up late at night as she discovered not enough sleep made her hungry. She learned to enjoy relaxing activities and gained an understanding of the relationship between exterior factors and fat loss.

Almost 3 months later, Andrea is still on the Lose Weight Here plan and continues to see results: She has dropped a total of 20 pounds and is now a size 4!

CHAPTER 1

LETTING GO OF TRADITIONAL DIET MODELS:

The Law of Metabolic Compensation

Remember playing tug-of-war as a child against an equally matched team? You pulled as hard as you could and the other side pulled back just as hard. You dug your heels in deeper, and they responded in kind. The battle continued until both sides became so tired they fell to the ground exhausted, with no clear winner. This is the game your metabolism is playing with you when you decide to diet using the traditional, status quo method: Eating Less, Exercising More.

We call it the Law of Metabolic Compensation, and it is the single most important element to understand about your metabolism. As you diet using the flawed Eat Less, Exercise More model, you set in motion a host of metabolic adjustments that lead to greater hunger, lower energy, increased cravings, and decreased metabolic rate. All of these changes are the way your metabolic thermostat tries to protect you from the stress of dieting.

Your body does this as a defense against what it perceives as starvation. Eat less, and you will have hormonal and brain chemistry changes that increase hunger and cravings. The body is intelligent, and its primary concern is defending its fat stores because it knows that once your body fat is gone, it can't survive. So it first increases hunger and cravings so you will eat more, then slows the metabolic rate so you will burn less. But remember the tug-of-war battle? Your metabolism is just as strong, if not stronger, than your willpower, and it becomes even more resistant the harder you work—to the point where it can halt or even reverse your dieting efforts.

You can certainly continue this tug-of-war game, but you likely won't win. Eventually, you will end up on the gym floor, a heap of exhausted rubble with a host of metabolic issues. This is metabolic damage, a state in which your metabolism inhibits weight loss and you also experience chronic fatigue, lack of motivation, mood changes, and digestive distress.

What happens when you let go of the rope in a tug-of-war battle? The other team goes tumbling helplessly to the ground. Letting go of the Eat Less, Exercise More dieting model is the first and most critical step in getting your metabolism back on track so you can attack stubborn body fat and trim down your shape. By working with the Law of Metabolic Compensation, you win the game of tug-of-war with your diet every time.

> **Letting go of the Eat Less, Exercise More dieting model is the first and most critical step in getting your metabolism back on track so you can attack stubborn body fat and trim your shape.**

Once you let go of traditional dieting, what do you do? There are two ways to create a calorie deficit and balance hormones for sustained fat loss. You can either Eat Less, Exercise Less (ELEL) or you can Eat More, Exercise More (EMEM). On this plan you'll do both, but at strategic and proven-effective intervals.

First, though, we're going to ask you to forget everything you know about weight loss and diets and start over. *Let go of the rope.* We want to reprogram your thinking. The way you've been addressing it so far, overall, is wrong. Reprogram your thinking and approach, and you will reprogram your lifestyle and see astonishing results. You won't gain back the weight you lose, and you'll be able to take off the really stubborn weight you've struggled with. You will reshape your body.

We're going to say it over and over: This isn't a one-size-fits-all approach. The

Can You Burn and Build at the Same Time?
The Myth of Metabolic Multitasking

To reshape your body, you have to both burn fat and develop muscle. The problem? Your metabolism isn't good at burning fat and building muscle at the same time. These two processes require completely different metabolic actions. They also require different hormonal signals. Building muscle requires insulin, while releasing fat for burning requires lower insulin. Burning fat and building muscle at the same time is the metabolic equivalent of patting your head and rubbing your tummy at the same time—it's not an easy task.

We call this the myth of metabolic multitasking. In reality, the body divvies up resources between burning fat (catabolism) and building muscle (anabolism). Your body wants to burn or build, but not both at the same time.

Understanding this aspect of metabolism allows you to fully harness its power. It's like trying to talk on the phone, cook dinner, and keep your kids from fighting with each other at the same time. You won't accomplish any of them well. Your phone conversation will be constantly interrupted. You'll burn dinner—or yourself. Your

kids may take it into the other room, but they'll continue fighting. To succeed, you have to give each task your full attention.

When you buy in to the myth of metabolic multitasking, you think that as you burn fat, you can simultaneously build muscle, but in reality, you'll be burning muscle too, and can wind up "skinny fat"—smaller than you were, but still flabby because you lost so much muscle. Likewise, if you try to build muscle in order to lose fat, you will add fat along with muscle and just look bulky. To burn fat and build muscle, the Lose Weight Here plan harnesses your metabolism's strengths at key times, so you'll alternate periods of burning fat and reducing your body mass with periods of muscle building and contouring.

Once you understand that metabolic multitasking is a myth and you begin to honor the Law of Metabolic Compensation, you'll start to burn fat from all over your body. The stubborn fat in troublesome areas will be burned off more quickly, too. Then, you can speed up the process even more by using the specific diet, exercise, and lifestyle techniques we'll be teaching you.

science applies to everybody, sure, but the exact formula you'll use to lose is very individual. Our science and plans will allow you to be a diet detective and tweak what we're offering you for optimum results. We are aware that this can be challenging because we all like black-and-white rules and certainty, but understanding that gray is everywhere will make you excel at doing the detective work. We call it structured flexibility. We'll provide the structure, you be flexible as you find the correct approach. We're not urging you to think like a "dieter"—we want you to think like a detective, sleuthing to create a path to the happiest, healthiest you. Before you lose any weight, you have to learn how to balance your metabolism. That's what we'll do first in this book.

Balancing your metabolism will:

◎ Curb hunger so you can naturally cut calories

◎ Bolster energy

◎ Control cravings for unhealthy foods

The end result: You'll finally achieve sustainable weight loss. We're busting the dieting myth here, and the proof will be the reshaping of your body.

CHECKING IN

Throughout this book, we're going to remind you to check in with yourself in a couple of ways.

Take AIM

You may feel like checking out when we talk about hormones, but understanding this information is vital to your success. To help you keep track of your hormones and their effects on your body, we break it down into the AIM process. Using it, you will Assess, Investigate, and Modify what you're doing until you find the key to losing weight. We'll arm you in the coming pages with the know-how to do just that, but you, as our partner in this, have to do the detective work.

Get Your HEC in Check

If your HEC—your hunger, energy, and cravings—is in check and balanced, you know your hormones and your metabolism are balanced, too—and no calorie counting is required. Hormones like insulin, cortisol, leptin, thyroid, and others have direct and indirect influence on your levels of hunger, energy, and cravings. When you are optimally producing and reacting to these hormones, HEC stays in check. If you do not produce the right amounts of hormones or lose the ability to respond to them (a condition called hormone resistance), HEC goes out of check.

MAJOR EFFECTS OF METABOLIC SLOWDOWN

Scientists have a pretty good handle on what might be happening when your metabolism slows down. There are many potential issues here, but we are going to cover what appear to be the three major effects that lead to this issue of weight-loss resistance and weight gain. One of them is probably going to surprise you.

Loss of Muscle Mass

Research shows that the basal metabolic rate (BMR)—the amount of energy you would burn in a day if you just sat around and did nothing—accounts for more than two-thirds of the calories burned in a day. Muscle tissues use more than half of the energy we burn at rest, so one of the best ways to offset the Law of Metabolic Compensation is to do everything in your power to gain or at least maintain muscle. To do that, protein and weight training are your best tools.

A study published in the *Journal of the American College of Nutrition* in April 1999 showed this effect. This study looked at a group of obese individuals who were put on a very-low-calorie diet and assigned to one of two exercise regimens. One group did aerobic exercise (walking, biking, or jogging four times per week), while the second group did resistance training three times per week and no aerobic exercise.

At the end of the 12-week study, both groups had lost weight, but the difference in the amount of muscle loss versus fat loss was telling. The aerobic group lost 37 pounds over the course of the study. Ten of those pounds came from muscle. In contrast, the resistance-training group lost 32 pounds. None of the weight they lost came from muscle. When the average BMR for each group was calculated, the aerobic group was shown to be burning *210 fewer* calories per day. The resistance-training group was instead burning *63 more* calories per day.

Hormonal Changes: Leptin and Thyroid

Whether you reduce calories or lower carbs, one of the first things that occurs in dieters is a beneficial change in the amount and/or sensitivity of the hormone insulin. Insulin also acts as a hunger hormone, so this change, while beneficial in the short run, is one of the first and earliest changes resulting in metabolic compensation. This causes increased hunger. Other hormones are also impacted. Cortisol, which is released when you're under stress, and ghrelin, which controls your appetite, are both elevated in spurts. This too causes increased hunger and cravings.

Along with the increased hunger and cravings comes the metabolic slowdown. This is most impacted by the metabolic hormone leptin. When a fat cell is shrinking and exposed to less insulin, leptin is also reduced. Low leptin excretion means increased hunger. Low leptin also means decreased activity of the body's two major metabolic engines, the thyroid and the adrenal glands. So as leptin decreases, your metabolism gets the signal to stop burning energy and instead start storing it.

Signs You Might Have Metabolic Damage

◎ Waist measurement of more than 35 inches for women and 40 inches for men

◎ An inability to control hunger and cravings

◎ High blood pressure (above 140/90 without medication)

◎ High-normal fasting blood sugar (higher than 95 to 100)

◎ Lipid abnormalities (high triglycerides and LDL cholesterol and low HDL)

If you do indeed have metabolic damage, the first step is to avoid the Eat Less, Exercise More approach. First you need to "fix the glitch" by avoiding the dieting mentality. Next you need to cycle the diet in a way that makes your metabolism more flexible and balanced and attacks stubborn fat, especially around the belly. Finally, you may require special supplements that aid insulin signaling and manage some of the symptoms. These might include alpha-lipoic acid, magnesium, B vitamins, berberine, and green tea extract. Talk with your doctor about the best approach to reversing your damage.

Leptin is considered by many to be the most important metabolic hormone in terms of setting metabolic output and weight regain. If you want to keep your metabolic rate up, you have to make sure your leptin level doesn't fall too fast, which we'll address later. The Lose Weight Here plan balances your leptin level and increases your metabolic rate. This effect varies substantially from person to person, with some people showing no effect from the brief period of overfeeding and others seeing a jump in resting calorie burn of several hundred calories per day.

Persistent Organic Pollutants

Persistent organic pollutants (POPs) are a group of hormone-disrupting chemicals that have a huge impact on metabolic compensation during dieting. These compounds have accumulated in your fat cells, and when fat is burned, they are released into your bloodstream in significant concentrations. The shocking thing about these compounds is that they do not come from your body. They are man-made chemicals that you eat, put on your skin, drink in your water, and inhale in the air; some examples are pesticides like DDT; compounds leached from plastics, such as bisphenol A, or BPA; and other industrial chemicals, like phthalates, and by-products of their breakdown, such as dioxins. Until very recently, no one understood how these compounds were involved in weight-loss resistance.

POPs are fat soluble, and thus become concentrated in fat. This means they're stored in the fat of animals that you eat, and also in *your* fat after you consume that animal fat. You can almost see this as a protective mechanism: If the POPs are in your fat cells, they can't do as much damage as when they're in your blood. So when they get in your body, you store them away in fat, where they biodegrade only very slowly. When you lose fat, however, they are released in significant amounts that can do more damage and slow the metabolism.

The bottom line is that when you lose fat, you *will* release more POPs—there is no way of getting around that, even though losing fat is a primary goal on the Lose Weight Here plan. But because this plan is very high in fiber (which binds to and helps remove toxins) and protein (which is required to make detoxifying enzymes) and is lower in fat (which means less POPs are coming in), it is the best tool we have to deal with this. We also try to do things in a way that mitigates the other two major causes of metabolic compensation: loss of muscle and hormonal changes.

POPs primarily impact the thyroid gland by decreasing its ability to make thyroid hormone, disrupting thyroid hormones once they are made, and speeding up the excretion of thyroid hormones. In other words, POPs damage thyroid function and drastically suppress metabolic function.

ACTIONS TO TAKE

We realize that this new information about metabolic compensation can be both exciting and confusing. Exciting because you finally have answers for why you regained all the weight and more from your last diet and why weight loss has been so difficult since then. Confusing, because what the hell do you do about it now?

The plan in this book outlines exactly how to deal with this issue, but before we get into the specific details we want to make sure you understand how the plan works and what went into it.

Much of the benefit comes from completely circumventing metabolic compensation. Here are the steps to beating metabolic compensation right up front.

Break the Diet Cycle

The best way to halt metabolic compensation is to avoid the Eat Less, Exercise More model to begin with. This is very easily accomplished by balancing your energy output and your calorie intake. In other words, if you are exercising less, then eat less too. If you are exercising more, then eat more. This is the way your favorite athlete gets that hard body we all admire. This approach also ensures you won't be losing muscle, which is a side effect of the ELEM approach that produces a "skinny fat" body: slim on the outside, but weak, mushy, and unhealthy underneath. The Lose Weight Here plan helps you avoid the bulked-up, swollen look, too.

Raise the Protein Content

In order to reduce fat, you must set your protein intake higher. Research shows that higher-protein diets, that is, ones exceeding the daily dietary reference intake of 0.8 gram of protein per kilogram (2.2 pounds) of body weight, help offset the decline in metabolic rate that occurs with dieting. In the Lose Weight Here program, our intention is to set the protein level at 30 to 40 percent of the total number of calories you eat, leaving approximately 30 percent for fat and 30 percent for carbs. Another way to think about this is to make sure you are getting at least 1 gram of protein per pound of body weight (if you want to gain muscle) or 1 gram per pound of muscle mass (if you are trying to just maintain muscle). If you are confused about body weight versus muscle mass, you can go to our online calculator at metaboliceffect.com/me-shape-calculator and it will do the calculations for you. The protein content of the Lose Weight Here plan is easily managed without a need to calculate a thing. You will see how easy this is once you get started with the plan. And for those who feel better knowing the numbers and formulas, we'll arm you with those tools as well—though we prefer that you not obsess and that you remember that your body is not a calculator.

Manage Your Carbohydrates

Carbohydrates are the new nutritional bad boys. If you listened to the anti-calorie and negative insulin dogma, you would think all you need to do to lose fat and keep it off is to reduce carbs to zero. That is a mistake that leads to metabolic compensation: Indiscriminately cutting calories or carbs can cause the exact things you're trying to avoid (fat storage and a weakened metabolism). The trick is to choose carbs that have higher amounts of fiber and water versus dry, sugar- and starch-rich carbs. This means getting most of your carbohydrate intake from nonstarchy vegetables, low-sugar fruits, and "wet carbs" like oats and beans instead of from breads and pastas. Remember, carbs—including starches—are not your enemy. The trick is to find the amount that keeps your HEC in check while not slowing down your fat loss—to find your unique tolerance level. And, while you may have heard that foods like rice and potatoes are the worst ones for fat loss, the high water content that comes along with the starch is extremely satisfying for many metabolic types. Including a small amount in your diet, rather than avoiding them altogether, is one of the key ways to reduce metabolic compensation and achieve lasting fat loss.

One way to assess whether a carb is helpful or hurtful is to understand how it impacts hormones. We'd like you to limit your intake of processed carbs, but if you do need to eat them in a pinch, you can use our hormonal carbohydrate calculator. It's simple: Calculate the hormonal carbs by adding the numbers of grams of fiber and protein and subtracting the result from the total grams of carbs. The lower the number, the better (shoot for foods that are a 10 or lower), with negative numbers being the best.

For example, let's look at a typical protein bar that has 24 grams of total carbs, 3 grams of fiber, and 10 grams of protein. Adding the protein (10 grams) and fiber (3 grams), we get 13 grams. When we subtract this from the total carbs (24 grams), we get 11 grams as this bar's hormonal carb amount. This number is higher than 10, so it is best avoided.

Nonstarchy vegetables like broccoli, spinach, and kale, as well as fruits like berries, are your best sources of helpful carbs. Unhelpful hormonal carbs that will not comply with this rule include starchy foods, especially dry starches—the ones that are devoid of water. These include things like cereals, breads, and pastas.

Below, we've listed some of the best carbs out there for weight loss and maintenance. Why do we deem them the best? Compared to other carbohydrates, they have more fiber and water relative to their sugar and starch content. They're also nutrient dense, which means there are more vitamins and minerals and phytonutrients (beneficial plant chemicals) per unit weight of the food.

Here's a list of some of the best carb-based foods.

◎ Apples

◎ Beans (high H_2O and fiber starch)

◎ Blueberries

◎ Broccoli

◎ Cabbage

◎ Carrots

◎ Cauliflower

◎ Chard

◎ Collard greens

◎ Grapefruit

◎ Green beans

◎ Green, leafy veggies, like lettuce and spinach

◎ Kale

◎ Oats (high H_2O starch)

◎ Oranges

◎ Pears

◎ Quinoa (high H_2O starch)

◎ Raspberries

◎ Rice (high H_2O starch)

◎ Strawberries

◎ Tomatoes

◎ White and sweet potatoes with the skin on (high H_2O starch)

Get the POPs Out

While we agree that fats have for too long been wrongly accused of being a main culprit in the obesity epidemic, there *is* an issue with high-fat foods that could be thwarting your weight loss: They often come loaded with POPs. As we discussed earlier, POPs wreak havoc on your HEC, affecting your thyroid function and drastically suppressing your metabolic function.

The number one way to avoid POPs is to avoid high-fat animal products. While it's true that POPs are in the soil and water and are sprayed on plants, plants do not hold on to POPs like animals do, since the pollutants are mainly fat soluble and plants contain little fat. The highest concentrations occur in the animals who eat the plants, who then collect the POPs in their fat cells.

So to minimize the effects of POPs until your body is able to eventually break them down and eliminate them, you first need to stop accumulating them. This means eating low-fat animal products, or if you are going to consume high-fat animal products, making sure they are organic to minimize your POP risk. You also need to be sure to eat lots and lots of vegetables. The antioxidants in veggies are protective against POPs and contain fiber that binds to POPs to help them leave the body. (When the liver gets rid of POPs, it does so by putting them in the gallbladder, where they are then released into the GI tract to be eliminated in the feces. Without adequate fiber ushering them out, they can easily be reabsorbed by the body.)

Making eating nonstarchy vegetables and lean protein sources your priority may be the best way to deal with the POP effect.

THE LOSE WEIGHT HERE RECAP

◎ The metabolism works like a thermostat—*not* a calculator.

◎ Beat metabolic compensation by giving up the Eat Less, Exercise More approach to dieting.

◎ Use the Eat Less, Exercise Less *or* Eat More, Exercise More approach to balance your metabolism and get your HEC in check.

◎ Increase protein intake to help you stay full, maintain your muscle mass, and minimize weight-gain rebound.

- Get most of your carbs from vegetables and fruits and find your unique tolerance for starches, focusing on the ones with high fiber and water content.

- Control the intake of POPs by reducing your consumption of fat from conventionally raised animals and ramping up your vegetable intake.

THE SCIENCE: *The Law of Metabolic Compensation*

The calorie counters want you to believe your body is a rudimentary calculator that only engages in adding and subtracting: Eat too many calories and/or use too few, and you gain weight. Add in more food and subtract out any exercise, and you gain weight.

What they don't tell you is that doing this causes the metabolism to respond in a way that increases hunger, lowers energy, increases cravings, and lowers metabolic rate. This is no small thing. This metabolic compensatory effect—the existence of which is undisputed in research on weight loss—means the harder you push on one end of your metabolism, the harder and more forcibly it will push back in the other direction.

Big and Individualized Effects

We humans can be a bit dense at times, and many of us forget this key fact: A solution that works in the short term but fails to work or even makes things worse in the long run is not really a solution. At best it is a waste of time, and at worst it amplifies the problem. Hence the high rate of diet failure and the reality that many dieters end up fatter than when they started.

Low-calorie dieting decreases the number of calories you burn per day by an average of about 300. But that is the average. For some, this effect is much larger, and for others it is less.

Many who are well versed in metabolism will immediately point out that if you lose weight, then of course you are going to be burning fewer calories because you have less body tissue. True. But what research shows, and our clinical experience validates, is that the reduced rate of metabolic output goes far beyond what would be predicted by loss of fat mass or muscle mass.

A person who weighs 180 pounds and diets down to 150 pounds burns much less energy than another person of the same height who also weighs 150 pounds but did not diet. Something about dieting causes an exaggerated slowdown in the metabolic rate that goes beyond what would be predicted based on tissue loss. And, as pointed out previously, along with this slowdown comes a strong and unrelenting biological sensation of a need for food. That is a recipe for weight regain.

You may have firsthand experience with this metabolic slowdown or have witnessed it happening to a friend or a family member. What you may not be aware of is that this effect can last for a long period after the diet is over, even after you have already gained back all the weight you lost or more!

We know from research that the compensatory effects of dieting last for months and possibly years and may damage the metabolism over the long run. Researchers publishing the results of a study in the *American Journal of Clinical Nutrition* wrote about it in "Long-Term Persistence of Adaptive Thermogenesis in Subjects Who Have Maintained a Reduced Body Weight." As clinicians who work with patients requiring weight loss for obesity, we can tell you with certainty that people can and do become weight-loss resistant and can develop some degree of metabolic damage. *Metabolic damage* is a nondiagnostic term that some of us in the weight-loss industry use to describe a set of functional disturbances. These disturbances include

severe metabolic compensations that result in a depressed metabolic rate, chronic fatigue, immune system suppression, and multiple hormonal effects, including suppressed thyroid function, adrenal stress, and loss of libido and/or cessation of menstruation.

Research has shown this is not an imaginary issue. As far back as 1975, researchers published a study in the journal *Lancet* that looked at the issue of weight-loss resistance. Twenty-nine women who claimed they could not lose weight were studied. The researchers, like many of us, assumed these women simply were not sticking to their diets. The researchers wanted to test their metabolisms by sequestering them in a house and controlling all the food they ate and the exercise they did. Each woman was put on a strict 1,500-calorie-a-day diet.

At the end of the 3-week period, most of the women were found to have lost weight. However, 10 women did not lose any weight, and one of the women actually gained weight. This makes two points very clear: First, metabolism varies from person to person. Second, compensatory reactions can suppress the metabolism so much that even very-low-calorie diets are no longer effective even in the short term.

Maryalice

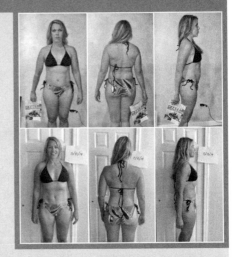

Maryalice hated living in her skin. She spent years running marathons and restricting and counting calories (she even kept spread sheets!). Eventually, her body hit what she called a "metabolic brick wall." She ran the Boston Marathon in 2008 and weighed more than she'd ever weighed. She didn't feel great and just kept putting on weight, which added to her emotional turmoil. She had zero energy.

Desperate, she tried everything from Reiki, to nutritionists, to diets, and even ended up on thyroid medication for hypothyroidism. The help from the medication was short lived as she quickly learned that her thyroid issue would have ups and downs and the medication would make her thyroid lazy. She came off the medication and focused hard on finding a solution. She worked with Dr. Jade for a few months and lost 17 pounds in 2012. Her energy was high and she felt like herself again. There were some hurdles that followed, including low iron, but once she went on the Lose Weight Here plan, she learned how to adjust to survive them. She pivots when she has to, changes things up when her body calls for it, and, in the end, is eating more than she used to. She's not hungry, and her HEC is in check.

CHAPTER 2

STARVE THE FAT, FEED THE LEAN:

The Law of Metabolic Multitasking

Y ou now know that the first step to changing your body shape and burning stubborn fat is breaking the diet cycle and avoiding the Eat Less, Exercise More approach. This helps you circumvent the Law of Metabolic Compensation, burn the fat, and maintain your results over the long run. This is required to correct the metabolic defect caused by dieting. You can think of this stage as "fixing the glitch."

The next step in the process is to cycle the diet. You'll spend some time in an Eat Less, Exercise Less (ELEL) state and then switch gears and move to an Eat More, Exercise More (EMEM) approach. This process allows you to focus all your attention on one area at a time, taking full advantage of your inability to burn fat and feed muscle simultaneously. You can think of the ELEL phase as starving the fat and the EMEM phase as feeding the lean.

Each of these two approaches will produce a different hormonal outcome. In the ELEL stage, you will be in a low-calorie-intake, low-insulin-secretion state. But because you will be combining that with higher amounts of protein, lots of walking, and a few weight-training sessions, your increased secretion of testosterone and human growth hormone (HGH) will also be working for you. This way, your muscles can be fed while your fat cells are starved.

HGH and testosterone are two of the few hormones that help the body multi-task better. HGH is best at burning fat, but it can also aid testosterone in building and toning muscle (though don't worry—it doesn't make you bulk up). Testosterone excels mostly at muscle building but also has some weak fat-burning properties. Together these hormones make the body a more efficient multitasker—the only problem is that there are very few things that raise these two hormones' levels together. Higher protein intake, weight training, adequate sleep, and longer periods between meals have all been shown to help generate more of one or both of these hormones. That is why the ELEL phase is structured the way it is.

KNOWING YOUR HORMONES

To understand how the Lose Weight Here plan is able to change the shape of your body, you need to know a little bit about how hormones work. This is important, because just as losing fat requires a calorie deficit and a certain hormonal balance, building muscle requires calories in excess and a different hormonal balance. We want you to understand exactly what is going on with your hormones and how they are working with your food intake to impact your overall shape and stubborn fat areas.

Certain hormones determine whether the body stores or burns fat. Many of them directly or indirectly control how hungry or full you feel, how predictable and stable your energy level is, and whether you will have cravings or not. While you can't "count" hormones the way you count calories, they impact feedback sensations that let you know if your hormones are balanced and your metabolism is functioning appropriately. Your hunger-energy-cravings (HEC) is one of the best indicators of whether you're on track. Remember, to achieve lasting fat loss you need your hormones to be balanced, and when they are, achieving a low-calorie state is almost effortless. Here are some of the hormones whose functions you should understand.

Fat-Burning Hormones

◎ **Human growth hormone** (HGH) is the building and burning hormone. It sends signals to be lean and muscular, and it works with cortisol and adrenaline to ensure that fat is burned rather than stored.

◎ **Thyroid hormone** is one of your body's fat-burning engines. It strongly impacts energy levels and is one of the major ways the body turns up the heat using its metabolic thermostat. It is the connection between thyroid hormone and leptin that may be most responsible for metabolic compensation. The thyroid gland is exquisitely sensitive to stress, including the stress of dieting. One of the major reasons you want to be very careful about decreasing calories by too much too fast or going too low carb is the negative impact each can have on thyroid hormone production. Much of what you will learn in this book is aimed at keeping the thyroid engine healthy and functional.

Hunger Hormones

◎ **Ghrelin and leptin.** Ghrelin impacts hunger from hour to hour, while leptin affects it from day to day. Ghrelin is also closely associated with cravings. As the ghrelin level rises after you go a long time without eating, hunger signals are sent to the brain. High ghrelin levels are very difficult to overcome using willpower alone. Eating protein and fiber and doing intense exercise can blunt ghrelin's message. Leptin is your fuel gauge hormone and is at the center of activity in your metabolic thermostat. Leptin tells the brain how much fat you have. If your brain loses the ability to hear leptin's signal (often a consequence of extreme dieting), you will keep eating as though you were starving. Leptin also regulates thyroid function. Leptin levels that are either too high or too low disrupt your metabolic thermostat, causing extreme metabolic compensation. This, again, is why extremely low-calorie and no- or very-low-carb diets almost always backfire. One of the reasons people become morbidly obese is because their bodies have lost the ability to receive leptin's message to stop eating and start burning.

◎ **Insulin.** There are two sides to insulin. On the one hand, insulin is a fat-storing hormone. High insulin levels often mean any extra calories will be stored as fat. Insulin also inhibits the body's ability to release fat, so you are less likely to burn fat in a low-calorie state. In other words, insulin often makes fat cells greedier, stingier, and more stubborn. The other side of insulin is talked about less—its ability to build muscle and control hunger. With the right approach (like this plan!), insulin can get HEC in check and create a tight, toned body. The trick with insulin and most other hormones is to achieve what we call the Goldilocks point—not too much, not too little, but rather just the right amount. Certain carbohydrates (starches, sweets, processed foods) are triggers for elevating the insulin level, and because of that, they are blamed for increasing fat storage and decreasing fat burning. But as you have just learned, having too little insulin might cause you to miss out on getting the muscles that make your body firm and tight, and satiety would be tougher to reach, as well.

◎ **Incretins.** Two of the most interesting hunger hormones are GIP (glucose-dependent insulinotropic peptide) and GLP (glucagon-like peptide). These two molecules are released by endocrine cells in the small intestine. As food travels through your digestive tract, these cells lining the small intestine sense the chemical composition of and even "taste" the food. When they do this, they release GIP and GLP to signal to the brain, pancreas, and other parts of the body how to respond to what is coming. The more sugar and fat you eat, the more GIP compared to GLP that is released. The more lean protein and vegetables you eat, the more GLP compared to GIP you get. One of the most important discoveries in obesity research in the last few years has been the way gastric bypass surgery reduces the number of GIP-releasing cells while increasing the proportion of GLP-releasing cells. We used to think that gastric bypass simply reduced the volume of food you can eat, but we now know that this happy consequence may be the major player reducing body weight and restoring metabolic function. You can think of GIP and GLP as twins. The chemistry of these two compounds is complicated, but a very simplistic way of understanding them is to see GIP as the evil, "fat-storing" twin and GLP as the good, fat-burning twin. If you can get more GLP signaling versus GIP signaling, you can mimic the impact of gastric bypass surgery without ever going under the knife.

Stress Hormones

◎ **Cortisol** is a two-sided coin as well—it can either help or hinder fat burning. You can think of cortisol as the 911 hormone: It is released anytime the body perceives a threat, whether that's emotional stress, food allergies, intense exercise, or missing a meal. Like insulin, cortisol behaves differently depending on the context in which it is released. Cortisol that is released in tandem with adrenaline, HGH, and testosterone, as is the case during exercise, becomes a positive and enhances fat burning. But when cortisol is released in the presence of high insulin, low testosterone, and limited HGH, as it is in the standard Western lifestyle, it acts as an unfriendly, fat-storing, muscle-burning hormone. The key with cortisol, as with insulin, is to understand how to manage it. Research tells us that cortisol and other stress hormones turn down the motivation centers in the brain while ramping up the reward centers. In other words, unbalanced cortisol levels are revealed by the sensation of cravings.

◎ **Adrenaline** is the gas-pedal hormone, and it is a close cousin of cortisol. When your metabolism is challenged, such as during exercise, adrenaline signals the body to begin burning fuel. A chain reaction then causes the release of other hormones like cortisol, testosterone, and HGH and the body goes into fat-burning mode. When adrenaline is released in someone who has high insulin and leptin levels but isn't exercising, it too can cause cravings and lead to loss of muscle.

◎ **NPY** (neuropeptide Y) is a brain hormone that is responsible for regulating hunger, but it is also released by the nervous system when you're under chronic stress. NPY causes fat cells to amplify in number and size and may be the long-hidden mechanism explaining why stress makes us fat. There seems to be a special relationship between cortisol and NPY. Chronically high levels of cortisol cause the nervous system to release more NPY and amplify its fat-storing effects.

Reproductive Hormones

◎ **Estrogen and progesterone** are not just reproductive hormones. There are receptors for both all over the body, including in brain, muscle, and fat cells. Their main function is regulating reproduction, but they also impact HEC and the ability to burn fat and build muscle. Estrogen and progesterone impact brain chemicals like GABA (gamma-aminobutyric acid, the most relaxing brain chemical), serotonin, and dopamine. This is one of the reasons HEC can get so out of check when women have their periods—estrogen and progesterone levels fall and cause brain changes that lead to moodiness, hunger, and cravings.

- **Estrogen** tends to keep women thinner all over, but leads to stubborn fat storage in certain areas, namely the hips, butt, and thighs. So estrogen is both a fat-burning and a fat-storing hormone. It also makes it easier for women to tolerate stress and better able to shape muscle while storing less fat. This is because it sensitizes the body to insulin and blocks the negative effects of cortisol.

- **Progesterone** makes women more likely to store fat and more likely to lose muscle because it opposes the action of estrogen. However, it does work with estrogen to block cortisol, so together, these two hormones create the desirable female hourglass shape.

- The Lose Weight Here plan will teach you how to use the natural fluctuations of these hormones to increase fat loss and enhance body shape. For women, the best time to follow the starve-the-fat approach is during the time of the month when estrogen is a little lower than progesterone. That is called the luteal phase of the menstrual cycle, and it spans the 2 weeks leading up to your period. The reason for this is that estrogen makes the stubborn fat in areas like the hips, butt, and thighs slightly more stubborn, so during the luteal phase you can take advantage of estrogen being a bit lower.

- During the follicular phase of the menstrual cycle, which is the 2 weeks after the start of a period, the estrogen level is higher. Because estrogen helps women shape muscles while minimizing fat gain, this is a great time to "feed the lean" by using the EMEM approach.

◎ **Testosterone,** like estrogen and progesterone, has effects all over the body. It helps shape and build muscle, and it creates the coveted V shape in the male physique. The story is a bit more complicated when it comes to women and testosterone, however: Higher amounts of testosterone compared to estrogen and progesterone thicken the waist and lead to more of an apple shape. This is why women who are greatly impacted by stress, have polycystic ovary syndrome, or are menopausal often gain more belly fat. So, when it comes to testosterone, it is not simply a matter of amount but rather of having the right balance.

HOW HORMONES REALLY WORK

You can think of hormones as your internal mail carriers; they are simply messengers. Whenever your body needs to make sure that some complex function takes place, like digestion or an adaptation to growth or a reaction to stress, it releases a hormonal messenger. The job of these messengers is to go tell cells how to respond.

Your body is never sending just one messenger at a time. It sends lots of messengers. Some tell the body to burn fat, some tell it to release sugar, others help control hunger and send the signal to build muscle. Your metabolism is constantly responding to multiple hormonal messages. When these messages are balanced and coordinated, hunger is suppressed, energy remains stable, cravings are subdued, and fat is burned while muscle is maintained. That's what you want and why focusing your attention on either muscle shaping *or* fat burning is critical. Trying to do both at the same time often confuses the messages and leads to poor results with either fat burning or muscle shaping.

HUNGER AND HORMONES

Let's step back for a second and look at one of the obvious big issues we face when we're struggling to lose weight: hunger. Hunger is both biochemical (influenced by hormones) and behavioral (influenced by habit). One thing to realize is that the behavioral component of hunger can be pretty powerful when you adjust the frequency of when you eat.

If you are eating five or six times per day and then switch to eating three times per day, you will experience hunger at all the times when you are used to eating. This is a learned response similar to the one in Pavlov's dog experiments, in which dogs fed shortly after the ringing of a bell learned to salivate and expect food anytime the bell rang, whether food was actually coming or not (and whether or not they were hungry). This is behavioral hunger; it is different from biochemical hunger, and humans are just as susceptible to it as dogs. This is actually a huge benefit of this new approach you will be learning. Most people never get a chance to *practice* mindfulness about hunger because they become overwhelmed by both biochemical and behavioral hunger. But because we will be controlling biochemical hunger during both the Eat Less, Exercise Less starve-the-fat phase and the Eat

More, Exercise More feed-the-lean phase, you will be able to practice overcoming behavioral hunger. With practice, you can train your body to not be influenced by your past behavior. This is all part of honing your detective skills and using what's called *skillpower* rather than relying on old diet habits and willpower.

What Your HEC Is Telling You

Use this cheat sheet to pinpoint what's causing your hunger, low energy, or cravings.

Hunger: When hunger is the issue, think leptin and insulin. They have either dropped too low because you have inadvertently restricted your food intake for too long or are too high because you have been eating too much of the wrong types of food. Control them by eating more foods that are higher in protein, fiber, and water. Then add wet starches or fat in small amounts up to your individual tolerance as a next step. To control behavioral hunger, drink water during typical mealtimes or eat water-based foods having negligible calories, like celery, lettuce, bell peppers, and cucumbers.

Energy: All the hormones affect your energy level, but insulin and cortisol are the big players since they dramatically impact blood sugar, and blood sugar balance is key to stabilizing energy. If your energy levels are low or unpredictable, first make sure you have not inadvertently put yourself in Eat Less, Exercise More (ELEM) mode. Make sure you are getting enough protein and that you have not cut carbohydrates or fats too low. If needed, add a few small snacks to your day. If this raises your energy level back up, then you will know it was a blood sugar issue. Try to avoid relying on stimulants like coffee and energy drinks, as these give you false energy and confuse your detective work. If abused, they can also add to any metabolic damage. A normal amount of coffee in the morning can be a beneficial and helpful thing for energy and health, but it should not be abused.

Cravings: Think stress and cortisol as well as habits and behavior. Take steps to lower your stress by prioritizing rest and recovery activities over stress-inducing activities. Physical affection, time with pets, leisure walking, hot baths, relaxing herbal teas, gentle stretching, massage, meditation, naps, restorative yoga, tai chi, relaxing music, and funny movies all lower stress hormones and can help beat cravings.

You're trained to eat when you're hungry, but if your hormones are out of whack, you are more likely to overeat when you're hungry. What we want you to do as you go through this process is to learn to read your hunger so you know what's working and what's not. We want you to be able to distinguish between biochemical hunger and behavioral hunger. You will also need to be able to discern hunger from cravings.

When you think you're hungry, is it because it's lunchtime or dinnertime and you're used to eating at that time? That is behavioral hunger. Or do you have a deep-burning, voracious hunger that is nagging at you from deep in your gut? That's biochemical hunger. If you pay close attention, you will see that behavioral hunger is less intense and more easily overcome. Biochemical hunger continues to reappear and gets stronger. Behavioral hunger often subsides as soon as you occupy your mind with something else.

We also want you to understand the difference between hunger and cravings. Hunger is felt in the gut: It is an empty, gnawing feeling. Cravings are felt in the head as a feeling of desire. So when you find yourself eating out of boredom, that is not hunger—it's a craving coming from the brain, not the gut. Cravings arise out of brain chemistry and habits.

You might be wondering how all of this relates to hormones and chemical interactions. While it is a bit simplistic, it is useful to think of cravings as related mostly to stress hormones like cortisol. In your brain, you have reward centers and goal-oriented motivation centers. When you are stressed, the stress turns down the goal centers, turns up the reward centers, and makes it more likely that you will fall back into habitual behaviors. This is not a good thing if you are trying to make a lifestyle change. When you think about hunger, it is most useful to think about insulin, leptin, and other hunger hormones.

There is one hormone that is associated with hunger *and* cravings—ghrelin. When you don't have food in your stomach, your ghrelin level will increase to tell your brain you're hungry. One way to remind yourself of this is to keep in mind that the words ghrelin and growl are similar. When you find your stomach growling, ghrelin is rising. You'll be feeling not only hunger but possibly also cravings at the same time. That may be ghrelin at work. This is important to understand. You may realize that skipping a meal or not snacking leads to this simultaneous hunger and craving, which then leads you to eat a large amount of the wrong foods in a short period of time. If this is the case, you will need to recognize it and develop strategies to deal with it. With the rising popularity of fasting and other eating strategies that decrease meal frequency, you need to be able to understand whether these tools work with or against your metabolic tendencies.

We realize that not everyone cares to know the names of the hormones involved and what they are doing. If you're one of these people, just remember this: If you are having cravings, think stress hormones and take the steps necessary to reduce the stress. If you are having true hunger, that requires a different approach, such as adding some snacks to your day to make sure your HEC is in check. Whenever you get confused about all this hormone and biochemistry talk, just go back to HEC. If HEC is in check, then your hormonal system is balanced. If HEC is not in check, you will need to do some tweaking.

THE BIOCHEMISTRY OF CRAVINGS

People often talk about cravings as though they were strictly biochemical. They are both behavioral and biochemical, and to fight them you need an approach that addresses both. Now you know a little bit about the behavioral reminders that can trigger cravings. You also know that following your routine continues to feed the cravings. But what about the biochemical aspect?

There are two very important biochemicals related to cravings. First is the chemical dopamine. It is the brain chemical of desire and floods the brain when you are seeking and finding pleasure—in this regard, it's a powerful motivator. The second is stress hormones. They play a key role because these hormones have been shown to shut off the motivating, goal-oriented parts of the brain while simultaneously activating the more primitive reward centers. In other words, stress hormones like cortisol may actually make you less motivated and more likely to seek out comfort foods, such as salty, sugary, and fatty foods. And this is why we often feel as if we're under a spell and are powerless to stop cravings when they hit despite the fact that we really, really, really want to stick to our goals. Stress hormones literally hijack the self-control center of your brain.

During a craving, you will feel a sense of want and desire (thanks to dopamine) along with a sense of anxiety or urgency (from stress hormones).

BREAKING HABITS

Cravings develop out of an expectation in the brain and are associated with the primitive reward centers of our brains. You can think of us humans as having one brain, but two minds. One of our minds is the unconscious mind, which is driven by habit, routine, and the avoidance of pain as well as the seeking of pleasure. The other mind is the conscious mind, which is driven by logic and is goal oriented and directive. Breaking your unconscious habits is the key to tackling cravings.

The series of events that defines a habit is often referred to as a habit loop. You can remember the habit loop by the three Rs (reminder, routine, reward). There is a reminder event followed by a repeated routine, which ends with a particular reward. And when this sequence (reminder, routine, reward) is repeated over and over, a craving develops, and that craving then ensures the routine will be repeated next time.

Here's an example. One of our patients, Sabrina, had a long-standing habit of sitting down with a glass of wine to watch TV every evening. This habit had become a real issue because it spawned a host of other issues that all negatively impacted her goal of body change: Watching TV was associated with wine, and both were associated with poor sleep. TV watching turned into staying up much later than she wanted to, and drinking wine turned into waking up repeatedly during the night. This then led to feeling fatigued and lethargic in the morning, which led to an inability to adhere to a morning exercise routine she had used to love. Her diet was impeccable, but her TV and wine habits were creating a domino effect that was keeping her stuck.

We discussed which habit was most detrimental (watching TV or drinking wine), and she thought that staying up late with the TV on was shortening her time in bed. So, we decided to change that first.

Sabrina *loved* TV. However, we asked her to limit her viewing each night to the one show she "had" to watch, and also talked with her about other things she loved to do. We found out she loved taking long baths—a perfect alternative to watching TV that allowed her to relax and did not prompt her to eat. This was a perfect start. We did nothing about the wine habit, as changing too much at once often leads to failure.

We started by overcoming the cues that would trigger her habitual actions. Previously, when her show was over, she got up and poured another glass of wine before coming back to the TV. Her new instructions were to get up after her favorite show, turn off the TV, pour another glass of wine if she wished, and go start a bath—taking care to light some candles and create a relaxing atmosphere. She could then drink the wine in the bath. We also asked her to pay close attention to old cues that told her to stay and watch TV. She had to make sure the TV was off before the next show's preview started or the intro music for the next show came on. She then needed to focus on the reward of having a relaxing time in a bath—something she loved—to prime the craving for that new routine.

This new approach not only worked for her, but also had an unforeseen outcome. She found that after having a glass of wine with her favorite show (which was on pretty early in the evening), she didn't feel the need to pour a glass for her bath. Almost immediately, she was drinking less wine and instead began a ritual of making herbal tea to have with her bath. She reported earlier times to bed, better sleep, and a more motivated and energetic morning of exercise. One small habit change led to a chain of positive effects that had an outcome opposite to that of her old habits.

THE FIX FOR CRAVINGS

Sabrina employed crucial strategies for overcoming a habit that was derailing her diet goals. Attack your own cravings using these steps.

Step 1: Pay Attention

Start noticing your cravings and paying very close attention to the environmental reminders that trigger them. Some of these are returning home from work, turning on the TV, sitting down at a restaurant, going out on a weekend night with friends, smelling doughnuts, seeing a friend eating a biscuit, having an emotional day at work or a poor night's sleep, and so on.

Step 2: Hack the Habit

Once you recognize the habit and the craving it creates, try to pinpoint the reward you are really after. Once you do, find a way to eliminate the trigger and/or change the routine so that the reward is the same but the craving that leads to it is different. Here is an example: Let's say you return home from work and you feel that combination of expectation, desire, and anxiety that tells you a craving has just been triggered. Now, identify the real reward that you are after. Is it relaxation? If so, instead of pouring a glass of wine and eating a wheel of cheese and a box of crackers (which in the end is anything but relaxing), draw a hot bath,

---

Five Metabolic Myths

◎ **Myth 1: The body is able to easily burn fat and build muscle at the same time.** For anyone other than those just beginning to exercise and those using anabolic hormones, simultaneously building muscle and burning fat is very difficult. It is best to focus on one, then switch and deal with the other.

◎ **Myth 2: All you need to worry about is calories.** Hormones directly influence how much we eat and what we choose to eat, so they play a key role in getting your body on track. Calories matter, of course, but they aren't the be-all and end-all of diet success, and focusing solely on calorie intake and expenditure is the main shortcoming of traditional Eat Less, Exercise More (ELEM) routines.

◎ **Myth 3: Hormones work in isolation and are either good, like human growth hormone, or bad, like cortisol.** The metabolism uses hormones to send messages about how to function elsewhere in the body. Hormones work in concert, and their ultimate action in cells is determined by the combination of hormones produced.

◎ **Myth 4: There is no good way to assess the balance of hormones without blood testing.** While testing is required to diagnose disease, biofeedback techniques like hunger-energy-cravings (HEC) can give a good subjective indication of metabolic hormone activity and balance.

◎ **Myth 5: The metabolisms of lean people and overweight people work in the same way.** Overweight and obese individuals often have multiple hormonal imbalances that make it more difficult for them to control hunger, stop cravings, and feel motivated to exercise. On this plan, you'll do the detective work to unlock your specific metabolic needs.

light some candles, and take 30 minutes away from the world. Practice this new routine over and over until a new craving develops.

Step 3: Balance the Brain

The brain is a hotbed of metabolic function and the origin of many of our cravings. When it comes to biochemical cravings, you want to try to achieve a balanced hormonal state in the brain. This means balance between the brain's major stimulating hormone, glutamate, and its major relaxing hormone, GABA. It also means achieving balance between dopamine (a hormone that helps us stay motivated, focused, and reward oriented) and serotonin (a hormone that helps us feel content, satisfied, and relaxed). There are several natural compounds that can be taken prior to getting cravings or even when cravings hit to stop them in their tracks.

◎ Cocoa powder (1 tablespoon in water)

◎ Branched-chain amino acids (5 to 10 grams)

◎ Tyrosine and 5-HTP (5-hydroxytryptophan) in a 10-to-1 ratio (1,000 milligrams of tyrosine and 100 milligrams of 5-HTP)

Each has unique properties that shut down cravings at the biochemical end. When combined with the behavioral component, you have a devastatingly effective solution for craving control.

Step 4: Assess

Cravings can be used as a biofeedback tool and are useful in helping you understand how your metabolism is functioning. Low blood sugar, too much or not enough exercise, missing meals or eating too frequently, sleep deprivation, and other lifestyle factors can impact cravings.

Always check in and ask yourself how your cravings have been. We have our patients assess their cravings, along with their hunger and energy, on a 1-to-10 scale (with 10 being strongest or highest). Obviously, you want the intensity of cravings to remain low, preferably less than 5. If this is not the case, then it is an indication that the diet and exercise regimen you're on is not sustainable. Understanding this allows you to manipulate several factors to correct it and turn short-term weight loss into long-term fat loss.

EVERYONE IS WIRED DIFFERENTLY

The commonly held belief that you will lose weight if you eat less and work out like crazy is simply wrong. In fact, it's a big pet peeve of ours that the health-and-fitness industry treats everyone exactly the same, especially when it comes to lean people and obese people. It can't be one-size-fits-all calorie cutting. You need to finesse everything we're telling you to make it work for and evolve with you. Being a diet detective and understanding your metabolism and hormones are the most important tools you have to get the weight off. The metabolisms of lean people don't act like those of overweight and obese people. Understanding this is critical if you happen to be obese.

If that's the case, you will struggle because your brain might not "hear" the signals sent by hormones like leptin and insulin, leaving you always unsatisfied and unable to feel full. Those nutritionists who say you should eat only when you're hungry aren't taking this biochemistry into account. The Eat Less, Exercise More model only makes the situation worse for you because it ensures that your hormonal chemistry will be unbalanced continuously, preventing you from hitting the Goldilocks point for those hormones. This is the reason you will need to follow an approach that cycles the diet and provides adequate protein, fiber, water, and other satiating macronutrients.

THE LOSE WEIGHT HERE RECAP

◎ Cycling the diet in a way that starves the fat (by eating less and exercising less) and feeds the lean (by eating more and exercising more) is the solution to this dilemma. Each of these approaches creates a unique hormonal state that, in combination with the other, balances calories and hormones in a way that enhances fat loss and muscle shaping.

◎ Understanding hormonal interactions and how they influence things like hunger, energy, and cravings is critical to understanding this new approach to body change.

Angela

At age 60, Angela was what she called a "metabolic slug." She worked out and ate well all day long, but, at night, she binged hard. She said her menopausal body steadily grew soft and puffy. She signed up for Metabolic Effect at the beginning of 2014, promised herself she would "get lean in 2014" and lost 14 pounds. She grew mindful of her eating and developed a strong and consistent workout routine.

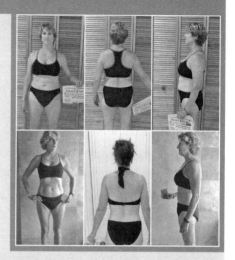

She started the Lose Weight Here plan and lost an additional 13 pounds and 8 inches, not to mention shedding the stress she lugged along. She won back time and her love for life. She knows what nutrition satiates her and what triggers her mindless eating. She's stopped obsessing and reads her body's signals so she knows when to rest and take a breather. Her body has more work to do, she says, but her mind-set is in a great place.

CHAPTER 3

TAKING AIM:

The Physiology of Stubborn Fat

I n order to jump into our program, there is another aspect of metabolism you should understand: the physiology of fat. You need to know how the body actually stores fat, why some fat tissue is more stubborn than others, and how fat burning really works.

Each type of body fat is unique. The stubborn fat around the hips, butt, and thighs can be targeted by combining diet, exercise, lifestyle changes, and supplements. But the fat sitting deep in the belly requires a completely different approach. To change your body, you must assess your unique physiology and metabolic tendencies, which determine where you store fat, how you burn it, and how you can replace that fat with lean, tight muscles.

THE SCIENCE OF FAT

Fat enters or leaves fat cells mainly due to the activity of two enzymes, lipoprotein lipase (LPL), which acts to store fat, and hormone-sensitive lipase (HSL), which acts to release fat. You can think of these two enzymes as big nightclub bouncers named Larry (LPL) and Harry (HSL). Larry stands outside and waits for his boss,

The Fat-Burning Process

In order for fat to be lost from a particular area, the following events need to occur.

◎ Fat needs to be released from a fat cell. This process of fat breakdown and release is called *lipolysis*.

◎ Fat needs to be carried through the bloodstream to another cell. Poor blood flow to an area means slow fat loss from that area.

◎ Fat needs to enter another cell to be burned. This process of fat actually being burned is called *lipid oxidation*.

It is important to note here that just because fat is broken down and released does not mean it will find its way to another cell and be burned. It could just be stored again, as is often the case for people who are very insulin resistant.

insulin, to tell him to let people in the club. This is analogous to a cell getting the signal to let fat in to be stored. The other bouncer, Harry, is responsible for kicking people out of the club. He takes orders from his boss, adrenaline.

Fat tissue has receptors that interact with certain hormones. These receptors are like the doors of the nightclub. Insulin holds the key and unlocks the front door for fat to come in, whereas adrenaline holds the key that unlocks the back door, where fat is shuttled out.

Here is where fat burning gets tricky. There are two types of receptors—"back doors"—adrenaline can use. One is bigger and can let more fat out, while the other is smaller and fat has to slowly squeeze its way out. The bigger doors are called beta-adrenergic receptors, and they speed up fat loss. The smaller doors are called alpha-adrenergic receptors, and they slow fat loss.

To keep this straight in your head, think *A* for *alpha* and *anti-burn* and *B* for *beta* and *burn*. In addition to having a direct impact on fat release, these receptors also impact blood flow. A body area that has more alpha-receptors gets less blood flow, and an area with more beta-receptors gets greater blood flow.

So what makes stubborn fat more stubborn? It has more alpha-receptors than beta-receptors.

Here is where the story gets interesting: Many types of hormones impact fat gain and fat loss. These hormones have this impact because of their direct or indirect effects on the enzymes (LPL and HSL) and receptors (betas and alphas) we just mentioned. Hormones that store fat or slow fat release tend to increase the number or activity of alpha-receptors and/or LPL. Hormones that stimulate fat release increase the number or activity of beta-receptors and/or HSL.

Certain hormones have a very straightforward impact on fat gain or loss. For example, insulin is a fat-storing hormone because it increases LPL activity and suppresses HSL activity. Insulin also impairs the normal functioning of beta-receptors and increases the activity of alpha-receptors.

Adrenaline speeds up fat release. It binds to beta-receptors, which increase HSL activity. But it also slows fat release if it instead binds to alpha-receptors. This is one of the reasons that stubborn fat, which has a higher concentration of alpha-receptors, can be so slow to respond.

Other hormones have more complex and overlapping activities. Estrogen increases the number and activity of alpha-adrenergic receptors. The fat distribution typical for women—predominantly in the lower body—is due to the impact of estrogen; women's subcutaneous fat, and especially their lower-body subcutaneous fat, is richer in estrogen receptors than that of men.

Thyroid hormone increases beta-receptor activity and blocks the activity of alpha-receptors. It therefore works against estrogen, making stubborn fat less stubborn. However, thyroid hormone is itself disrupted by estrogen (that's one of the reasons women have more issues with their thyroids than men do).

Is your head spinning yet? Don't worry, it will all make sense soon. Here are a few takeaways regarding stubborn fat in general and some hormonal effects to keep in mind.

◎ Stubborn fat has more alpha-receptors and fewer beta-receptors.

◎ Stubborn fat stores more fat and releases less of it under the influence of insulin.

◎ Stubborn fat has less blood flowing through it.

◎ Hormones that increase HSL activity and/or inhibit LPL activity stimulate fat release.

◎ Hormones that decrease HSL activity and/or stimulate LPL action encourage fat storage.

◎ Stubborn fat is stubborn not because it can't be released, but rather because it releases fat much more slowly than less stubborn fat does.

◎ The sex steroids (estrogen, progesterone, and testosterone) bind to receptors in fat tissue and play important roles in HSL and LPL activity, as well as impacting the numbers and activity levels of alpha- and beta-receptors.

FAT VERSUS STUBBORN FAT

So what exactly do we mean when we say *stubborn fat*? You probably know where your own "trouble spot" is, but what's the scientific explanation? Well, basically, we store fat in a variety of places in our body.

There is fat stored just underneath the skin. We call this *subcutaneous fat*. This is the squishy stuff that hangs over your belt and appears lumpy. Then there is fat we store deep inside the torso, around our organs and under our abdominal muscles; another name for the internal organs is the *viscera*, so this is called *visceral fat*. This is the stuff that gives many men that large, protruding belly. You can't pinch this stuff—it's compacted and fairly hard. Finally, there is fat stored in and around our muscles. This is called *intramuscular fat*. If you look at a piece of beef at the butcher's, all that marbling around the muscle is similar to our intramuscular fat.

Female Stubborn Fat

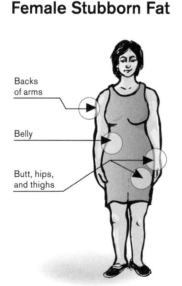

Backs of arms

Belly

Butt, hips, and thighs

Male Stubborn Fat

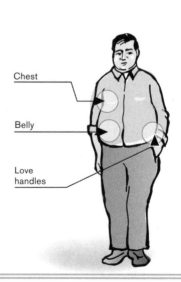

Chest

Belly

Love handles

The most stubborn fat on the body is the fat under our skin, the subcutaneous fat. And female subcutaneous fat is more stubborn than male subcutaneous fat. The most stubborn fat in the majority of women is lower-body subcutaneous fat, around the hips, butt, and thighs (you may know it as your beloved saddlebags, thunder thighs, or bubble butt). The most stubborn fat on men is the subcutaneous fat of the lower abdomen (often called the love handles). Now do you feel like you can relate or understand what we mean by that stubborn fat?

Remember:

◎ Subcutaneous fat is far more difficult to lose than visceral fat.

◎ Subcutaneous fat is stubborn because it is more reactive to insulin, has a lower blood supply, *and* has more alpha-receptors.

◎ Visceral fat is less stubborn because it has more beta-receptors, gets greater blood flow, and is less reactive to insulin.

◎ Subcutaneous fat in the lower body of a woman has significantly more alpha-receptors and fewer beta-receptors than the lower-body fat of a man.

◎ The places on men where fat is most stubborn are the lower belly and love handles.

◎ The places where the fat is the most stubborn on women are the saddlebags, inner thighs, butt, and lower belly.

◎ Another reason stubborn fat is stubborn is because it has more alpha-receptors, which results in poor blood supply.

◎ Stubborn fat is impacted directly or indirectly by many different types of hormones. These hormones have varying effects on the activity of HSL and LPL as well as on alpha- and beta-receptors.

FEMALE LOWER-BODY FAT: BUTT, HIPS, AND THIGHS

This area of a woman's body naturally stores more fat and is more stubborn about releasing it. This is due to the physiology of fat, as we already discussed: It has more alpha-receptors and fewer beta-receptors.

Many women think they can "outrun" their lower-body fat by exercising, but controlling this area is really more about controlling the diet. The only way to

Female versus Male Belly Fat

Female belly fat is more about stress. Women with high waist-to-hip ratios (bigger bellies), whether overweight or underweight, have been shown in research to be more stress reactive. This means that dealing with female belly fat is less about diet and exercise and more about stress management. Which is good to know, because when food and exercise are taken to the extreme, they, too, can become a stressor. This is why we often say that a woman with stubborn belly fat that does not respond to diet and exercise would be far better off spending an extra hour in bed than an extra hour on the treadmill.

◎ The stress that causes female belly fat leads to a unique hormonal situation where testosterone and cortisol are high while estrogen is low.

◎ Eating less and exercising less (ELEL)–"starving the fat"–which is phase one in our plan, may be the best approach to use for female belly fat since it is focused on relaxation and recovery. If you are a woman with a large amount of belly fat, you may choose to stay in this phase for much longer.

Male belly fat is a bit different and, unlike female belly fat, it is helped rather than hurt by having more testosterone. In males, belly fat is more an issue of having lower testosterone and higher cortisol and insulin levels. Male belly fat will respond to both ELEL (starving the fat) or EMEM (Eat More, Exercise More) (feeding the lean). For male belly fat, carbohydrate intake modification is key. Carbohydrate intake should not be too low or too high–both extremes lead to hormonal imbalance. Too low means increased cortisol and slowed loss of belly fat; too high means too much insulin and slowed loss of belly fat. Once again, the Goldilocks concept applies.

target this fat and get it to burn at the same rate as that in the rest of the body is to make sure you are controlling secretion of the hormone insulin and using the natural fluctuations in estrogen level to your advantage.

The best way to control cortisol is also the best way to control insulin: Use the Eat Less, Exercise Less approach. But women really wanting to attack female lower-body fat should pay particular attention to when they start the first phase of the Lose Weight Here diet—the ELEL phase. Since estrogen increases the activity of alpha-receptors, the ELEL approach should be done during the late luteal and early follicular phases of the menstrual cycle: the week before and week during their period. This is the time of the month when the estrogen level is the lowest and release of this fat is most likely to speed up.

Part of your detective work is to learn how this is done. Later, we will go into more detail on the diet, exercise, and supplement tactics to use to attack female lower-body fat, but here we wanted to make sure you understand the mechanism controlling this unique area of stubborn fat. Once you've cycled through the protocols and entered the maintenance phase, we'll offer you even more targeted and specific approaches for attacking your trouble spots.

THE LOSE WEIGHT HERE RECAP

There are three types of fat:

◎ Subcutaneous fat—the stubborn one

◎ Visceral fat

◎ Intramuscular fat

◎ Stubborn fat is unique physiologically because it is far more reactive to insulin and has greater numbers of alpha-adrenergic receptors.

◎ Stubborn fat in certain areas of the body varies and there are definitely gender differences due to the impacts of hormones like estrogen, progesterone, and testosterone.

◎ To beat stubborn fat, alternate the Eat Less, Exercise Less and the Eat More, Exercise More phases to circumvent the body's natural aversion to simultaneously burning fat and building muscle.

Luis

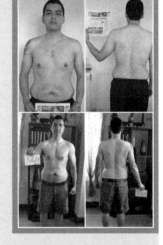

Luis describes himself as a chunky kid, despite having been into sports growing up. Ridiculed by friends and family about his weight, Luis used his personality to muddle through and not let the jokes get him down. By the time he turned 18, he hit a funk, became depressed, and gained 100 pounds in less than 12 months. He was so upset about the weight and the stretch marks that he never left his house. At his father's urging to find a solution, he spent years working at his weight by trying every diet and form of exercise out there, yo-yoing his way through them all.

His wife introduced him to Lose Weight Here. At first, he was hesitant and worried he'd disappoint his wife by failing at yet another diet program. But 11 pounds and 2 percent less body fat later, he didn't. He lost the weight, and he gained a lot of time back too. He'd been doing classes and working out like a maniac, all while working two jobs. Not anymore. He no longer eats sugar, and he's been able to use the time to set personal goals. He's saved money because he eats at home more and he's got renewed energy.

His biggest lesson learned from Lose Weight Here: You don't have to suffer and starve to get results.

CHAPTER 4

THE DIET DETECTIVE:

The Law of Metabolic Individuality

Before we let you dive in and get started, we'd like to make sure that we've truly redefined the word *diet* for you, so that you no longer consider eating less and exercising more to be a legitimate diet. Now that you understand how destructive that methodology is to your metabolism and how destined you are to fail by using it, we want you to embrace your individuality and be aware that that old approach violates what we call the Law of Metabolic Individuality. Subtle differences in each person's physiology and metabolism make them different from everyone else. Understanding that each of us is as different on the inside chemically as we are on the outside physically is key. In addition, we each have psychological predispositions that make us react differently to stressors, foods, people, and exercise. And we also have huge variations in our personal preferences.

The truth of the matter is that there is no such thing as the perfect diet. Those who are successful at balancing their metabolisms and losing weight don't *discover* a diet; rather, they create the right diet for themselves. They don't follow a particular diet; they build a lifestyle that fits their unique metabolism, psychology, and personal preferences.

Diets don't address any of these differences. Dieters almost always fail because they have this very wrong belief that there is a perfect diet out there somewhere that they just need to find.

The truth of the matter is that there is no such thing as the perfect diet. Those who are successful at balancing their metabolisms and losing weight don't *discover* a diet; rather, they create the right diet for themselves. They don't follow a particular diet; they build a lifestyle that fits their unique metabolism, psychology, and personal preferences so that it's sustainable for life. And they do this by using a methodology and mind-set very different from what's typically found in diet books. They do it through trial and error and the basic framework we're providing you with here.

PRACTICE AND MASTERY

We humans are funny; we realize in most other worthwhile endeavors that mastery is a process, not a recipe. In other words, if you want to be a great pianist, there is no procedure you follow from start to finish that provides a linear and predictable outcome. The process is individual and has ups and downs, peaks and valleys, with great triumphs followed by frustrating failures. And all along the way we learn, practice, and master the steps until we become proficient. This process of practicing to achieve mastery is an individual journey we all must make, and it applies to dieting, too.

From this moment on, you have to realize *you can no longer approach your body-change goals with the mind-set of a dieter.* We are going to teach you how to do that. What is beautiful about escaping the dieting trap is that you will never again be confused about your metabolism and what you are doing wrong. Instead, you will slowly learn to understand your body and its needs better than anyone else on the planet.

A DETECTIVE, NOT A DIETER

So how do you create the diet and lifestyle perfectly suited to you? You become a detective. Get rid of the dieter in you. A detective does not solve a problem by following a predefined recipe. He or she learns to master the skill of observation and lets the clues gathered guide him or her to the solution.

A skilled detective can also develop an uncanny ability to see past the wrong assumptions and myths the rest of us fall prey to. Good detectives simply see things more clearly and fully. Whereas dieters see things in only black and white, detectives see all the shades of gray, and rather than shrinking back from the complexity, they embrace it.

Becoming a detective means that you first need to put aside all your preconceived notions about rules of exercise and food. Here are a few examples.

◎ Carbs are the devil.

◎ You must always eat breakfast.

◎ You should only eat certain foods at certain times.

◎ Eating less and exercising more is the route to weight loss.

These types of diet biases will be your worst enemy if you hope to finally break through the diet trap and see lasting change. These types of beliefs have done nothing but confuse people for decades. In the 1980s, we were told that fat will kill you. Then we were told that carbs will make you fat and kill you. Now we are told fat is the dietary savior from heaven. Some people are also now trying to convince you that protein is what will really kill you. If you have these biases and refuse to give them up, you will be in for a long struggle with diet confusion and misery.

There is only one diet rule that is true: Do what works for you.

As a detective, you are searching for the perfect mix of ingredients that will make you feel great, easily help you lose weight, and improve your laboratory blood values and vital stats. If eating jelly beans all day gives you that kind of health and vitality, then that is what your body needs, no matter what anyone tells you. We doubt, of course, that you'd have much success with the jelly bean diet, and we also understand that this idea of "finding what works for you" can be extremely nerve-racking. You might be asking, "How the hell do you do that?"

There is only one diet rule that is true: Do what works for you.

Well, good detectives become masters of a few essential tools. Once you are armed with the tools, it's up to you to use them over and over again until you master them.

STRUCTURED FLEXIBILITY

Since we crave certainty, people usually find the calorie-counting model alluring. We like the simplicity of seeing our bodies work like calculators. It makes sense and gives us a sense of certainty and confidence. The problem? The model is wrong.

So how can you have the certainty you need, while at the same time being free to explore the mystery of your metabolism so you can create your own diet? Structured flexibility, that's how.

In this book, we are going to provide you with a plan. However, this plan is not meant to be followed like one presented in any other diet book traditionally would be. It is meant to be a starting point only, a blueprint of sorts. It provides the structure you will need in the beginning, but then you must deviate from it by tweaking, adjusting, and adding and subtracting elements. The plan provides the structure, and your experimenting and detective work will create and build in the flexibility. Your goal: Discover exactly what works for you and achieve the amazing results we know this approach can deliver.

KEEP HEC IN CHECK

Detectives need tools. The first tool we will ask you to utilize is your hunger-energy-cravings (HEC). We have already described HEC, but now we want to discuss it in the context of being a detective. Your body is constantly providing feedback in the form of sensations. These sensations are directly impacted by hormones and give you a sense of whether you're in metabolic balance or not. Remember, hormonal balance is one of the two requirements for sustained fat loss.

In a sense, you can *count* your hormones by subjectively analyzing sensations like hunger, energy, and cravings. By keeping your HEC in check, you will also be keeping your metabolism in balance.

The beautiful thing about HEC is that it fluctuates constantly based on what you eat and how you live. If you eat the wrong things, your HEC will be out of check. If you exercise for too long or too intensely, your HEC will go out of check. If you are sleep deprived or stressed, HEC is impacted. Puberty, pregnancy, the menstrual cycle, menopause, male andropause, and aging all impact HEC. In fact, anytime your metabolic thermostat readjusts, your HEC may be impacted. HEC is your magnifying glass into the workings of your metabolism. It allows you to analyze your metabolic processes from hour to hour, day to day, and week to week. If HEC is in check, then you know you are on the right track. If it is not, that's an early alarm bell warning that you are in dieting mode again and will soon suffer the consequences.

Using HEC

At the end of each week, make a note of each of the parameters separately. What was your hunger like? Was it high or was it low? To better quantify it, give it a subjective score from 1 to 10, with 1 being a low level of hunger and 10 meaning very high hunger. You want to have a hunger score of less than 5.

Do the same thing for energy. Was it high, stable, and predictable? If so, you might rank it a 9 or 10. Or was it very low, unpredictable, and unstable? If that was the case, you might rank it a 3 or 4. You want an energy score of 6 or better.

Cravings are scored the same way. Frequent and unrelenting cravings get a high score and absent or weak cravings get a low score. Cravings, just like hunger, should be at less than 5.

You don't have to write the scores down, but do at least make a mental note of them. If any one of the three is out of check, then your HEC as a whole is out of check. Once you have this assessment, you can investigate, like a detective, what may have had a positive or negative influence and then take steps to adjust your approach to take this into account. This is a critical tool for creating the perfect plan designed for you, by you.

Steps to Get HEC in Check

HEC is a very individual thing, so this is an area where you will need to evaluate your need to follow exact rules. We are going to tell you the steps we take with our patients to get their HECs in check. We suggest that you follow this structure exactly at first. But then, as you get the hang of mastering HEC, feel free to tweak and adjust it to your needs—that's the structured flexibility concept that you will need to master as you take up this new approach to dieting.

Hunger, energy, and cravings are all impacted by blood sugar. The two best approaches to slowing the digestion of food, and therefore the absorption of sugar, is to include higher amounts of protein and fiber. Protein and vegetables help balance blood sugar and provide plenty of bulk to fill you up. Because they have less fat and starch, they also have very few calories. In other words, they give the one-two punch of low calories and hormonal balance, the ideal formula for fat loss.

If adding more protein, fiber, and water to your meals does not get your HEC in check, the next step is to add either starch or fat. We suggest that you try adding fat first. If that does not work, then add starch but take out the fat. Still not the right formula for you? Try combining a small amount of fat and starch. Finally, give more frequent eating a try by adding snacks. Give yourself a few days between changes to assess the outcome.

Once you dive into the plans, this will become very simple to implement, but as an overview, the steps to take when your HEC is out of whack are:

1. Add more protein, fiber, and water (such as lean protein and veggies).

2. Add fat.

3. Add starch and subtract fat.

4. Add starch and fat.

5. Add one or two snacks between meals.

How much of each should you add? As you've probably guessed, it varies for each person. We will suggest amounts, but ultimately the amount will be up to you. To start, though, think in bites.

◎ **Protein and fiber:** Consider adding 5 more bites of each. That is approximately 4 ounces (20 grams of protein) and probably 8 ounces (1 cup) of vegetables.

◎ **Starch:** Consider adding 3 big bites of starch. That is about ½ cup (15 grams of carbs).

◎ **Fat:** Consider adding 1 extra bite—1 tablespoon (10 grams of fat).

Remember, your metabolism is unique to you, so these are just our rough guidelines to provide you with a basic structure. You have to stay flexible in your approach and be open to trial and error. It might sound daunting at first, but you will soon find your ideal diet. It may take time to figure it out, but when you do, it will make a huge difference and before you know it, it will become completely intuitive and automatic, turning you into a skilled detective able to adjust your metabolism on the fly. There is no greater skill to have in mastering your metabolism and blasting your stubborn fat.

Your Shape Change Means Results

HEC is an amazing tool, but it is not the only one you will use. You also need to be able to properly assess the results you get with any change in your diet, exercise regimen, or lifestyle. Most people get this all wrong. Weighing yourself tells you very little about the type of weight you have gained or lost. You might be losing fat, or you could be losing muscle. In the game of shape change, muscle is what gives you tone. You definitely do not want to lose it.

This is why measuring what your body is made of is critical. You want to know how much fat versus muscle you have lost or gained. But even that is not enough. When you are trying to attack stubborn fat, you need to know if your shape is changing in the right proportions. That says much about how you will look after doing all of this work.

The only way to effectively know if you are burning stubborn fat is by experiencing a shift in your shape. When your apple or pear shape begins turning into a V shape (for men) or an hourglass shape (for women), you know you are successfully burning stubborn fat.

Your tools for measuring body composition are a scale and a tape measure. In doing this work for 20-some years, we have tried every tool there is to measure fat

---

Hot or Not?

Researchers have actually studied body shape and attractiveness. Their findings have revealed that the healthiest body shapes, and those that both men and women prefer in terms of attractiveness for themselves and others, are the hourglass shape for women and the V shape for men. Coincidently, these shape measurements also tell you everything you need to know about how successful you have been at burning your stubborn fat. An apple- or pear-shaped woman will never achieve the hourglass shape unless she burns the stubborn fat from her belly, hips, butt, and thighs. A man will never achieve the V shape unless he can successfully get rid of those stubborn love handles.

versus muscle: weight scales, skin calipers that pinch your fat, and those fancy scales that give you a body-fat reading. But we found that none of these tools adequately assesses body shape in the way that is required to attack stubborn fat.

How to Measure Shaping Success

Men will measure their waist-to-chest ratio, while women will measure both their waist-to-chest ratio and their waist-to-hip ratio to assess their body shape. For the hourglass shape, women want the waist-to-hip ratio—what we call the *pear point*—to be symmetrical with the waist-to-chest ratio, which we call the *apple point.*

Both of these numbers should be between 0.6 and 0.9. The closer a woman gets to 0.7 and the closer the two numbers are to being the same, the more pronounced her hourglass shape and the better she is at losing stubborn fat. For men, the waist-to-chest ratio should be less than 0.8, with 0.77 being the number typically preferred by those who are romantically interested in men.

What is beautiful about using this method of measurement is that it takes into account the individual shapes and sizes of all humans. Whether you are thin, tall, short, or stout, you can still achieve the hourglass or V shape. In fact, you can be overweight and still be an hourglass. The assessment to make is: When you lose fat, are you maintaining the hourglass shape or becoming more of a pear or an apple? If you are already an apple or pear shape, is that shape morphing into the hourglass shape or simply becoming a smaller, more pronounced, and mushier apple or pear shape? This tells you everything you need to know about how stubborn your stubborn fat is. Are you successfully unlocking it to the same degree that you are in the rest of your body?

If your pear point—the waist-to-hip ratio—starts drifting further away from 0.7 and closer to 0.6, you know you are not successfully reaching the stubborn fat in the hip, butt, and thighs. If your apple point—the waist-to-chest ratio—starts moving away from 0.7 and closer to 0.8, then you know you are not successfully getting at the stubborn belly fat.

How to Measure Yourself

◎ Always measure yourself at the same time of day and under the same conditions. We suggest doing this first thing Friday morning, before eating or drinking anything.

Female Measuring Points

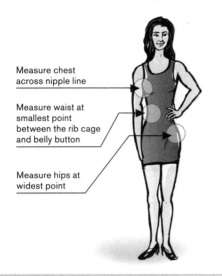

Measure chest across nipple line

Measure waist at smallest point between the rib cage and belly button

Measure hips at widest point

Male Measuring Points

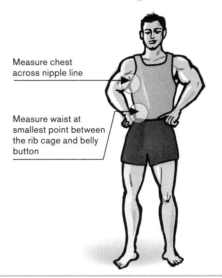

Measure chest across nipple line

Measure waist at smallest point between the rib cage and belly button

Calculate

Waist-to-chest ratio (apple point):
Normal is 0.6 to 0.9 and 0.7 is optimal

Waist-to-hip ratio (pear point):
Normal is 0.6 to 0.9 and 0.7 is optimal

Hourglass shape = both waist-to-hip and waist-to-chest ratios are approximately equal

Calculate

Waist-to-chest ratio (apple point):
Normal is 0.7 to 0.8 and 0.77 is optimal

V shape = waist-to-hip ratio below 0.8

◎ Measure your chest across the nipple line (women, do this while wearing a bra).

◎ Measure your waist at the smallest point above your belly button, but below the bottom of the rib cage.

◎ Measure your hips at their widest point (women only).

◎ Weigh yourself without wearing clothing or shoes. (Women should wear a bra.)

WHEN YOU ARE NOT BURNING FAT

If you are assessing your shape and doing your measurements but not losing fat, you need to figure out why. Again, this is a very individual process. It is impossible for us to predict what unique mix of diet, exercise, and lifestyle will be right for you.

For ease, you can use our online shape-calculating tool at metaboliceffect.com/me-shape-calculator. We will do the calculations for you and send them right to your e-mail.

What we can tell you is *never, ever* use exercise to burn extra fat or get yourself moving. It simply does not work in the long run and will almost assuredly cause weight-gain rebound because it almost always throws HEC out of check. Do not make the mistake of trying to put weight loss on a metabolic credit card. Stubborn fat is burned in the kitchen. *Always make your adjustments with your food.* Using exercise in this way is one of the most important negative habits to break as you make the transition from dieter to metabolic detective.

Remember: We will give you structure by helping you understand what we do in our clinic, but you need to allow yourself to be flexible within this process, and even to break our "rules" if it's required. We suggest you start by using this exact process and tweaking it as needed.

Here are the steps to follow. Give yourself a week (or at the least a few days) with each stage. If the first approach does not work, go to the next approach. Keep in mind that these adjustments should be made only after HEC is in check. If HEC is not in check, balance it first.

1. Cut back on starchy foods at each meal.

2. Move all your starch intake to one meal only (the best choice is breakfast, dinner, or in a postworkout snack).

3. Cut back on fat.

4. Eat less frequently.

5. Search for and eliminate trigger foods (we'll address these in the coming chapters).

6. Start closely monitoring calorie intake.

The first two steps are usually the most powerful. We refer to them as finding your carbohydrate tipping point. This is the amount of starch, the type of starch, and the timing of starch intake that keeps HEC in check and helps you burn fat. Don't make the classic dieter's mistake of cutting starch out completely. The only time you should completely eliminate carbs is if doing so keeps your HEC in

<table>
<tr><td colspan="5" align="center">**Carb Cutbacks to Consider**</td></tr>
<tr><td>3 big bites</td><td>*or*</td><td>15 grams of carbs</td><td>*or*</td><td>½ cup</td></tr>
<tr><td colspan="5" align="center">**Fat Cutbacks to Consider**</td></tr>
<tr><td>1 bite</td><td>*or*</td><td>10 grams of fat</td><td>*or*</td><td>1 tablespoon</td></tr>
</table>

check and helps you burn fat. But we have seen very few extremely low-carb dieters accomplish that over the long run.

THE FAT-BLAST FORMULA: AIM

The third tool in the detective's tool kit is the process of analyzing HEC and your shape-change results. This is the most critical process for a detective—it's where the metabolic mystery is solved. It is how you know whether you need to adjust your approach and what direction you should head in.

To use this tool, remember the acronym *AIM* that we have discussed: assess, investigate, and modify.

◎ **Assess** by checking in on HEC and your shape-change results.

◎ **Investigate** the results. Was your HEC in check? Did you lose fat, and in the right places?

◎ **Modify** by asking: Do I need to increase foods rich in protein, fiber, and water to stop hunger? Or add in a little more carbs to stop cravings?

What are the steps you need to take? This process teaches you.

Potential Outcomes

There are four potential outcomes from this process, each having a particular follow-up approach to consider.

Outcome One

Assess: HEC in check, fat lost, and shape changed in the right places

Investigate: This is the holy grail of body change. You have solved the mystery of your metabolism and effectively unlocked your stubborn fat. You now have the opportunity to understand how your metabolism functions. It may be that you stumbled upon this result, or it could be that trial and error predictably led you to this point. Either way, make a note of how you arrived here and all the elements involved, from diet and exercise to lifestyle and mind-set.

Modify: Don't make the two critical mistakes that many people make: Do *not* try to speed things up by pushing harder on your metabolism. Do that, and you are more likely to push yourself right out of this balanced state. Do not start looking for another way. We humans are funny; when we find something that works, we often promptly stop doing it. Your job now is to practice, practice, practice.

Outcome Two

Assess: HEC in check, fat *not* lost and even gained

Investigate: With this outcome, you know you are doing something correctly, because you have solved one side of the equation: hormonal balance. You know this because your HEC is in check. But your fat-loss results either are not happening or are heading in the wrong direction. Surprisingly, this situation is not as bad as you think. The fact that your HEC is in check means you are operating from a place of strength and your metabolism will be able to tolerate you pushing on it a little harder without overreacting. Since HEC is in check, you can focus on the two biggest components of your diet that increase calories and unbalance hormones—fat and starch. We will tell you the steps we take with our patients, but remember, you are your own detective. Therefore, it is up to you to filter this through your preferences and what you know about your body.

Modify: Here are the steps to follow.

1. Cut back on starchy foods at each meal.
2. Move all your starch intake to one meal (the best choice is breakfast, dinner, or a postworkout snack).
3. Cut back on fat.
4. Eat less frequently.
5. Search for and eliminate trigger foods.
6. Start closely monitoring calorie intake.

Outcome Three

Assess: HEC not in check, but fat lost and shape changed in the right places

Investigate: You may think this is a desirable state, but it is the classic dieter's trap. It is alluring because you are getting some short-term results. But the fact that your HEC is out of check tells you that you are in a state of metabolic compensation and will soon experience the fate 95 percent of dieters do: yo-yo weight regain. If you are really unlucky, you will actually end up fatter after these positive short-term results. And if you are extremely unlucky, you will damage your metabolism and wind up with more—and more stubborn—fat.

Modify: In this scenario, you need to get HEC back in check.

1. Add more protein, fiber, and water (such as lean protein and veggies).

2. Add fat.

3. Add starch and subtract fat.

4. Add starch and fat.

5. Add one or two snacks between meals.

Outcome Four

Assess: HEC not in check and fat not lost or gained

Investigate: You've got some detective work to do! By now we hope we have drilled into you that the first order of business is to get HEC in check. Once that is done, then you can start working on burning fat. In this scenario, you should be careful to take it one step at a time. Get HEC in check first, then work on fat loss second.

Modify: Here are the steps. Notice how this is a combination of HEC strategies and fat-loss strategies. One hint here is that adding more protein, fiber, and water-filled foods is often the only strategy required. This increases food volume and lowers calories by displacing high-calorie foods, which often creates the best of both worlds in one fell swoop. Always take this step first.

1. Add more protein, fiber, and water (such as lean protein and veggies).

2. Cut back on starchy foods at each meal.

3. Add one or two snacks between meals.

4. Move all your starch intake to one meal (the best choice is breakfast, dinner, or a postworkout snack).

5. Adjust fat intake up or down.

6. Look for and eliminate trigger foods.

7. Track calorie intake.

THE LOSE WEIGHT HERE RECAP

If you are like most people, this chapter and the concepts presented in it probably have your head swimming from a mix of excitement and feeling overwhelmed. That is normal. This is a brand-new conceptualization of and approach to dieting for almost all of our patients. It is also extremely liberating, providing you with a blueprint and structure and giving you the tools to create the approach that's right for you.

Remember, you are as different from others on the inside, chemically, as you are on the outside, physically. A one-size-fits-all approach to dieting does not and cannot work. What does work is learning the process of discovering, practicing, and mastering the ins and outs of your own metabolism. This book gives you the master plan for making this happen.

Monitor your HEC. We typically wait 7 to 14 days for fat-loss results to show. But you can make changes much more quickly as far as HEC is concerned. Also, remember that in the beginning, you should follow the outline we give you in a systematic fashion. It's okay to keep the training wheels on and get some miles under your belt before going it alone.

Now it is time to get into the plans. We want to caution you at this point not to slip back into dieting mode. You are now a detective. We are going to provide a starting point with the in-depth plans presented in the chapters to come. But be warned: The plans are purposely flexible and designed specifically to avoid the dieting trap of rigid rules and defined guidelines.

We are going to give you an airtight structure with which to start, but using the steps we've given you, we fully expect you to take responsibility for altering the approach to suit your metabolism, psychology, and personal preferences.

Let's get started.

Katherine

Having spent most of her life overweight, in 2010, Katherine worked hard to lose 45 pounds. She wanted to lose more but could never quiet get rid of that extra stubborn fat and eventually started to notice the weight she'd lost was creeping back. Menopause didn't help, nor did all the years she had spent on extreme diets.

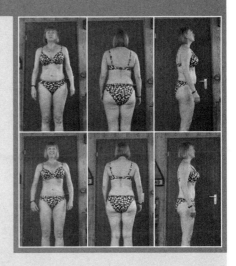

She started with Metabolic Effect and built muscle and got strong, then she jumped into Lose Weight Here to see what she could do. Instead of 5 days a week of working out, she focused on relaxing and walking 10,000 steps a day. She cycled her diet and lost 11 pounds quickly. More important, she shrunk— shedding inches in all of her trouble, stubborn spots. She measured herself and was shocked to learn she weighed more than she had at her lowest weight 20 years ago but was much, much smaller over all.

Measurements and photos were helpful to Katherine on her journey, and she learned to ride the scale's ebb and flow, focusing more on how her clothes fit than her weight. She learned how critical sleep was to her efforts and walking too. Mostly, she found the plan sustainable and grew confident she'd reach her goal eventually.

Part II

The Lose Weight Here Program

Kristina

Stress took its toll on 58-year-old Kristina. Her metabolic issues were 14 years in the making. Desperate to keep her weight low, she had accepted the low energy that came with a 600- to 700-calorie day. When she saw a coach for help, she tripled her calories and didn't modify her exercise. In addition, she was always taking care of everyone else, never herself. Her reward for the emotional wear-and-tear and advice from a health professional: 30 extra pounds.

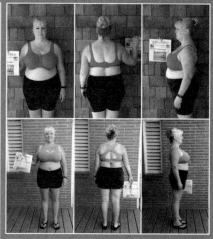

Lose Weight Here helped her understand metabolic function more fully. Her first big step: letting go of the eat less, exercise more mentality. She also ditched any notion that one size fits all. With the simple tools she learned, she dropped 14 pounds and shed 9 inches in 12 weeks. More important, she figured out how to weather the assault of the latest and greatest diet plans to find what worked for her.

CHAPTER 5

STARVE THE FAT PHASE:

Eat Less, Exercise Less

W hen a sculptor starts a new figure, she removes large pieces from an unshapely mass of clay to reveal the general shape of the figure she has visualized in her mind's eye. Similarly, this fat-blasting stage of the Lose Weight Here plan removes fat from the entire body. It's called "starving the fat." To do so, you'll Eat Less, Exercise Less (ELEL). This phase is best thought of as a means to repair your damaged metabolism and starve your fat—getting rid of those large pieces of clay—without feeling starved.

In this phase, you will:

◎ Eat less food and consume fewer calories

◎ Exercise less frequently

◎ Eat three meals a day

◎ Eat fat and starch sparingly

◎ Fast for 12 hours every night after dinner

◎ Weight train only twice a week

◎ Eliminate intense cardio workouts

Why Fast Overnight?

In the 3-2-1 protocol, we ask you to go 12 hours without eating, creating equal time for your system to go without food.

Fasting overnight has many benefits. It can:

◎ **Give the digestive system a breather.** In essence, we are giving the metabolism time off from digestion, assimilation, and storage, giving it more time for recovery, repair, and accessing stored fat.

◎ **Give the immune system a break from any food allergies and sensitivities.** If you experience food sensitivities and/or allergies, a less frequent eating pattern will be more beneficial and less stressful to the metabolism.

◎ **Allow the body to access its stored calories and fat.** Many people eat so frequently that they never give their bodies a chance to start accessing the fat stores. The longer you go without food, the more likely you are to dip in to your fat stores for energy.

◎ **Aid in staving off behavioral hunger.** Many people are ruled by behavioral hunger. Overnight fasting allows people to practice mindfulness when they are hungry, lessening the chance of a behavioral hunger episode.

This formula creates the unique metabolic environment discussed in the previous chapters that reverses metabolic damage and burns fat fast. You will follow the ELEL plan for 2 weeks—using biofeedback to assess, investigate, and modify the plan to keep your hunger-energy-cravings (HEC) in check. For these 2 weeks, think 3-2-1: You'll follow a simple 3-2-1 eating plan and a 3-2-1 exercise plan.

 ## ELEL AT A GLANCE

The 3-2-1 Eating Plan

◎ 3 meals a day

◎ 2 meals are protein based and sugar- and starch-free

◎ 1 meal is a regular 3-2-1 meal and should include starch

The 3-2-1 Dinner Plate

What do we mean by a "regular" meal? This meal should follow a 3-2-1 pattern on your plate: 3 parts vegetables, 2 parts lean protein, and 1 part starch or fat.

The 3-2-1 Exercise Plan

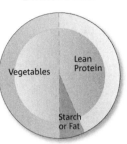

The 3-2-1 Dinner Plate

◎ 3 rest and recovery (R&R) activities per week

◎ 2 traditional weight-training sessions per week

◎ 1 to 2 hours of leisurely walking (about 5,000 to 10,000 steps) on all or most days

---

Diet Detective

WINE AND ALCOHOL

You'll notice that we've included one glass of red wine in our sample week. Alcohol can cause issues for your weight-loss and metabolism-balancing efforts: It is high in calories (second only to fat), and, like fats and carbs, is metabolized to acetyl CoA. When acetyl CoA is around in high amounts, the body sees no reason to burn other fuels, so when you drink, you are more likely to store your calories as fat rather than burn them.

You may wonder, then, why we are not telling you to avoid alcohol completely. The truth is, it may be necessary for you to avoid it, but we have also seen people have wine almost nightly and be able to attain and maintain a lean, healthy body. The trick is to know what does and does not work for you. As we have said before, you have to honor your own metabolism, psychology, and personal preferences. Small amounts of alcohol can certainly be a part of some people's fat-loss formula. Whether it is for you or not will take some detective work.

Understanding interactions between certain foods is critical. If you want a glass of wine with dinner, don't eat starch and fat with your meal. Make an effort to never combine the three. For instance, have a piece of fish, a plate of veggies, and either a glass of wine *or* half a sweet potato, but not both. Experimenting is key and our goal is to provide you with structured flexibility. We're just giving you the blueprint.

The 3-2-1 Week

A sample week on this plan might look like this.

DAY	MEAL 1	MEAL 2	MEAL 3	EXERCISE	R&R
Monday	Protein smoothie or high-protein and vegetable meal	Protein smoothie or high-protein and vegetable meal	Small salad with a vinegar-based dressing, 2 cups broccoli, 8 ounces grilled chicken, ½ sweet potato	1–2 hours of leisurely walking (about 5,000–10,000 steps)	Hot bath with Epsom salts
Tuesday	Protein smoothie or high-protein and vegetable meal	Protein smoothie or high-protein and vegetable meal	8 ounces grilled salmon, 2 cups green beans, 2 cups broccoli, ½ cup cooked rice	Weight training and 1–2 hours of leisurely walking (about 5,000–10,000 steps)	
Wednesday	Protein smoothie or high-protein and vegetable meal	Protein smoothie or high-protein and vegetable meal	Grilled beef fillet steak, 10 asparagus spears, ½ baked potato	1–2 hours of leisurely walking (about 5,000–10,000 steps)	30-minute nap
Thursday	Protein smoothie or high-protein and vegetable meal	Protein smoothie or high-protein and vegetable meal	Mexican grilled chicken and vegetable fajita with ¼ cup cooked rice, ¼ cup beans	Weight training and 1–2 hours of leisurely walking (about 5,000–10,000 steps)	
Friday	Protein smoothie or high-protein and vegetable meal	Protein smoothie or high-protein and vegetable meal	Large chopped salad with grilled chicken, 1 cup vegetable soup		Restorative yoga class
Saturday	Protein smoothie or high-protein and vegetable meal	Protein smoothie or high-protein and vegetable meal	Grilled halibut, mixed vegetables, jasmine rice, one 8-ounce glass red wine		Watch funny movie
Sunday	Protein smoothie or high-protein and vegetable meal	Protein smoothie or high-protein and vegetable meal	Bunless Bison hamburger with lettuce, tomato, and onion, 1 cup baked sweet potato fries	1–2 hours of leisurely walking (about 5,000–10,000 steps)	

Meals 1 and 2: Protein-Based and Vegetable Meals

Protein Shakes

We like to tell people to use protein shakes because they are consistent, measurable, and easy to manipulate if adjustments are needed. They lay the groundwork for a perfect case study in being a diet detective. The shakes usually provide exactly what you need biochemically, and therefore allow you to more clearly understand your behavioral eating issues. If you're used to eating six times per day, you will entrain that eating response and be hungry—you guessed it—six times per day. If you then change your eating pattern to three times per day, like we're suggesting, you're probably going to be hungry at the other times you normally eat, at least for the first week. Your body is used to the habit of eating more often. Give your body at least a week to adjust. If after that point your HEC still isn't in check, you will need to start doing some detective work to figure out how to control it.

Break the Habit Loop and Stop Behavioral Cravings

Take note of your behavioral eating needs versus your biochemical ones. The habit loop goes like this: reminder, routine, and reward. The reminder might be coming home from work. Then you set down your keys and other things. The routine has begun. Maybe you plop down on the couch, pour yourself some wine, and turn on the TV. That's the reward. Doing it over and over makes you develop a craving for it. Simply walking in the door triggers the routine and reward. The only way to break it is to interrupt the routine. Here are a few suggestions for doing so.

- Go to the gym after work.
- Stop at the coffee shop to catch up on some e-mails.
- Go outside and do some gardening.
- Take a bath and have some herbal tea.

The Water Debate

The water issue is tricky, and you will hear all sorts of advice regarding water. Some people will tell you not to drink too much with meals because it will "dilute your digestive enzymes." Others will tell you that the hunger and thirst mechanisms get confused, and that when you feel hungry, it actually might be an indication that you are thirsty. Still others will tell you to force water down your throat every chance you get. What we will tell you is to use water in a way that works for you. Stay hydrated with water, but don't go crazy; just check to make sure you are drinking enough to make your urine a very light yellow.

The best use of water is to control HEC—drink plenty with meals to fill up. We have found no objective information that suggests water intake at all interferes with digestion; in fact, it more likely helps. Also, in this phase, while you're eating fewer meals, to help circumvent behavioral hunger, drink a large glass of water during the times you would normally have a meal but now are not.

Making Your Protein Shakes

The protein shakes on this plan are truly simple: Just combine 20 to 50 grams of protein powder with unsweetened almond or coconut milk, water, or low-fat dairy milk. The best way to enjoy the shake you're drinking is to find a protein powder you really like. If you don't like the taste of it, you won't use it. Obviously, as natural health practitioners, we prefer you stick to ones with more natural ingredients. In fact, we prefer that you use real food instead of shakes, but we realize that is impractical for many due to our busy lifestyles. If you have any food sensitivities, thyroid issues, or autoimmune conditions, you may want to consider a dairy-free brand since dairy foods can be an issue for some people. Dairy is a great, healthy food for most, but many others experience hidden negative effects from it, partly because it can produce too much insulin in some people, slowing fat loss. It is also a common allergen.

Once you've done some trial and error, you'll find a protein powder you like. Then you can experiment with the liquid you mix it with. Try unsweetened

Choosing Protein Powder

When choosing a protein powder, be sure to check the label. Try to use a protein that yields a negative number when you subtract the combined protein and fiber total from the total carbohydrate grams. Many products claim to be "protein shakes" but are actually mostly starchy and/or sweet smoothies with more carbohydrates than protein. That is *not* what you want. Choose a brand that delivers at least 20 grams per serving. The number of grams of protein plus the number of grams of fiber should exceed the carb grams in the shake.

Here are a few protein brands we and our patients like:

◎ **Metabolic Effect's Protein Meal Replacement:** You can get this on our site at metaboliceffect.com/proteinshakes.

◎ **Isagenix:** You can order this through our site at metaboliceffect.com/proteinshakes.

◎ **Vega Sport:** Find this online and at Whole Foods or Vitamin Shoppe.

◎ **Hemp Force:** Find this at Whole Foods.

◎ **PlantFusion:** Find this at Whole Foods.

◎ **Jay Robb:** Most health food stores carry this line.

◎ **BioTrust Protein:** You can order this through our site at metaboliceffect.com/proteinshakes.

almond or coconut milk or water to start. (We recommend avoiding dairy here, too, because those who have an issue with it often don't even know it.) These options are also low in fat and starch, allowing you to engage in your detective work to understand how the macronutrients may be impacting you. Using almond or coconut milk rather than water also tends to increase the viscosity of the shake a little, making it more substantial (which you might find that you like). You can certainly use dairy milk if you prefer, but keep in mind: It may add more calories and increases the potential for allergy issues. If you do use milk, consider trying a low-fat version (1% or 2%) at first to be able to detect the HEC impact of fat versus protein.

The 5-4-1 Approach for Cravings

While we prefer that you do not snack, we know some of you may experience hypoglycemia if you don't. If you're in the first phase and you continue to feel light-headed or unable to focus or you have persistent uncontrollable cravings at night, an easy modification is to divide up each shake and split them into two meals to create a 5-4-1 approach.

◎ 5 meals per day

◎ 4 of those 5 meals are small protein shakes spaced every 2 to 4 hours

◎ 1 regular-balance meal including protein, fat, and carbs at night

You're not eating any more doing it this way, but you are eating more frequently. While this is not the ideal approach for most, some will need to make this modification.

Protein Meals

We suggest shakes for the sake of convenience, and also because they provide a consistent macronutrient profile (the same protein, carb, and fat content each time). They are quick and easy for those who don't have time to prep and cook full meals, and they take thinking out of the equation.

However, a high-vegetable, protein-based meal that's low in fat and starch is preferred over shakes. If you'd rather put together your own protein-based meals—say, because you need to chew to really feel full—you do have options. If protein shakes aren't for you, aim to eat 20 to 50 grams of protein through food sources at those meals, with little to no starches or fats.

Make sure you're not considering legumes and nuts to be protein in this protocol. They do have protein and will keep your body from becoming protein deficient, but they are mostly sources of fat and starch. Many vegetarians and vegans eat mostly starch (we call them carbotarians or starchatarians because rather than eating mostly vegetables, they eat mostly grain foods).

Here are a few solid-food, protein-based meal options:

◎ **Omelets.** Our favorite is a 4-egg omelet with ½ cup each of raw tomatoes, spinach, and mushrooms. We are big fans of the yoke—one of the healthiest foods on earth, so feel free to keep some or all of them in. If you feel you need to do detective work on your fat intake, though, egg whites can serve the purpose as a pure protein source.

⊚ **Meat and veggies.** We like a 4- to 8-ounce chicken breast with a side salad or 1 to 2 cups of your favorite veggie (such as green beans or broccoli).

⊚ **Protein-based soup.** If you have the time, it is a good idea to cook up a big vat and eat from that over the week. We use a slow cooker to make our favorite: Place 6 boneless, skinless chicken thighs, 1 head chopped kale, 1 large chopped onion, 1 small bag (about 16 ounces) precut, prewashed baby carrots, 9 to 12 cloves crushed garlic, and 1 tablespoon chopped fresh or dried rosemary plus sea salt and ground black pepper to taste in a slow cooker. Cook on low for 8 hours. Divide into small containers and store for the week for an easy meal you can quickly heat up for lunch or dinner.

Convenience Salad

Another great way to get your first two protein-based meals of the day is to have what we call a convenience salad. This is any meal that is all protein and vegetables, and it couldn't be easier to create: Just keep the protein, double the vegetables, and subtract the starch and fat. This easy formula allows you to create a meal anywhere: at an Italian restaurant, when you're ordering Chinese food, at a party or barbecue—wherever. For example, if you order a sandwich or burger, ask for extra lettuce, tomato, and onion and throw away the bun—you now have an ELEL-friendly lunch.

Meal 3: Your 3-2-1 Meals

While your third meal of the day will follow the 3-2-1 formula (3 parts vegetables, 2 parts protein, and 1 part starch), it also allows you the most flexibility. We've provided plenty of options for this meal starting on page 69, but feel free to get creative. Swap fish, chicken, steak, pork, or a vegetarian meat replacement for the specified protein. Replace the starch with any other high-fiber wet starch you desire or have on hand (such as beans and legumes, sweet potatoes with the skin, or quinoa).

Tummy Trouble?

Protein and vegetables are the toughest foods to digest, absorb, and assimilate, which is one of the primary reasons they're called for during this eating phase. Translation: They control hunger-energy-cravings (HEC). Many longtime dieters will find that the metabolic damage they have done has caused weak digestion. If this is the case for you, making you feel gassy or bloated after you eat, try these tactics.

◎ Make sure your vegetables are well cooked.

◎ Increase protein content in meals slowly over time.

◎ Use a good-quality digestive enzyme product to help your body break down and digest these foods. If you would like to compare the one we use in our clinic with your favorite over-the-counter brand, you can check out our version here: metaboliceffect.com/product/metabolicenzymes.

Spice Things Up

Eating properly doesn't mean resigning yourself to rubbery steamed chicken and boring plain lettuce. We encourage you to spice up your food to make it more enjoyable. In fact, some spices are actually tremendously beneficial to your system. Here are some ways to add flavor—plus nutrition—to your meals.

◎ Vinegar is great for your digestion and can decrease the blood sugar and insulin response when added to high-starch meals. Use a vinegar-based dressing on your salad.

◎ Cinnamon, like vinegar, decreases blood sugar and the insulin response to starches. We love adding it to our shakes in the morning.

◎ Saffron adds a unique flavor to savory dishes—and it helps blunt hunger.

◎ Cocoa powder reduces cravings. Mix it with water to curb cravings and reap its many health benefits for the heart and brain.

◎ Turmeric is great for reducing inflammation.

◎ Ginger decreases inflammation and aids digestive function.

◎ Garlic is a great source of sulfur, which aids in detoxification. It is also antiviral and antibacterial.

◎ Onion powder, like garlic, can help in detoxification and also contains the antioxidant quercetin.

◎ Lemon pepper seasoning has some mild metabolism-boosting effects.

◎ Rosemary is great for the heart and blood pressure.

◎ Thyme contains the antioxidant thymol.

◎ Basil is an excellent heart-healthy herb. It also acts as an antioxidant and even has some antimicrobial effects.

◎ Oregano also has excellent antioxidant properties. We use oregano oil in our clinic as a natural antifungal.

◎ Coconut amino acids are a great soy-free replacement for soy sauce for those who are sensitive to soy foods.

 ## THE 3-2-1 RECIPES

Sage-Rubbed Chicken

1 teaspoon dried sage	¼ teaspoon sea salt
1 teaspoon garlic powder	4 chicken legs or breasts
¼–½ teaspoon ground black pepper	1 onion, finely chopped

Preheat the oven to 375°F.

Mix together the sage, garlic powder, black pepper, and salt in a small bowl and generously rub the mixture all over the chicken, getting under the skin if possible. Arrange the chicken in a glass baking dish and sprinkle with the onion.

Bake, uncovered, for 45 to 60 minutes. Pair with Brussels sprouts and ½ cup cooked rice.

SERVES 4

Per serving:
260 calories, 31g protein, 3g carbs, 1g fiber, 13g fat

Stuffed Peppers

Stuffed peppers are a great way to eat multiple servings of vegetables. They are low carb (but you have the option to add a grain if you want), filling, and incredibly versatile.

4 bell peppers (any color)

1–2 tablespoons extra virgin olive oil

1 small onion, chopped

3 cloves garlic, crushed

1 pound ground meat (try turkey, bison, or chicken)

½ zucchini, chopped

½ cup shredded carrots

2 cups tomato sauce (any low-sugar pasta sauce will work; amount can vary according to preference)

Dried oregano to taste

Dried basil to taste

Dried parsley to taste

Red pepper flakes to taste

Sea salt to taste

Ground black pepper to taste

Brown rice or another grain or pasta, such as quinoa or orzo (optional)

Your favorite shredded cheese (optional)

Preheat the broiler. Clean and halve the bell peppers lengthwise and remove the seeds. Place the pepper halves in a shallow baking dish, cut side down, and coat with cooking spray. Broil for about 5 minutes on each side or until starting to blacken slightly. Remove them from the broiler. Reduce the oven temperature to 350°F. Meanwhile, heat a sauté pan over medium to high heat. Add the oil. Cook the onion and garlic until slightly soft. Add the meat and cook until no longer pink. Add the zucchini and carrots, cooking for 2 to 3 minutes. Add the tomato sauce and mix thoroughly. Add the oregano, basil, parsley, red pepper, salt, and black pepper, making sure to test the flavor as you go. Stuff each bell pepper half with the meat and vegetable mixture. Bake for 15 to 20 minutes, or until heated through. Top with the cheese, if desired, during the last 5 minutes of baking.

SERVES 4

Per serving:
320 calories, 27g protein, 21g carbs, 6g fiber, 15g fat

Fat-Loss-Friendly Meat Loaf

1 tablespoon extra virgin olive oil

½ cup finely chopped onion

½ cup grated zucchini

3 cloves garlic, minced

1 egg

2 tablespoons dried Italian seasoning

2 teaspoons finely chopped fresh parsley

Pinch of sea salt

Pinch of ground black pepper

7 ounces (half of 13.5-ounce can) coconut milk

2 tablespoons ketchup (organic is preferable)

1 pound ground bison or grass-fed beef

1 cup almond meal

Heat a sauté pan with the oil over medium-high heat. Add the onion, zucchini, and garlic and cook, stirring frequently, until soft. Set aside and let cool. Combine the egg, Italian seasoning, parsley, salt, black pepper, coconut milk, ketchup, ground meat, and cooled veggies. Add the almond meal and mix until well combined. Place the mixture in a loaf pan coated with nonstick cooking spray and bake at 325°F for 35 minutes or until cooked through.

SERVES 4

Per serving:
530 calories, 30g protein, 12g carbs, 4g fiber, 41g fat

Simple Chili-Spiced Shrimp

1 pound small shrimp	2 scallions, chopped
1 tablespoon lime juice	Ground black pepper to taste
½–1 teaspoon chili powder	Sea salt to taste
2 cloves garlic, chopped	Hot sauce to taste

Peel and rinse the shrimp and place them in a large bowl. Add the lime juice, chili powder, garlic, and scallions. Marinate for 10 to 15 minutes. Heat a sauté pan over medium heat. Coat it with cooking spray. Pour the shrimp mixture into the pan and cook, stirring frequently, until lightly browned. Be careful not to overcook the shrimp. Season with salt, black pepper, and hot sauce to taste.

SERVING OPTIONS

Shrimp Tacos: *Place a small amount of the shrimp mixture on a corn tortilla and top with queso fresco, chopped fresh cilantro, avocado, sautéed bell peppers, and sautéed onions.*

Shrimp Taco Salad: *Place the shrimp mixture on a bed of spinach and add grilled veggies, salsa, and avocado.*

SERVES 4

Per serving:
90 calories, 16g protein, 3g carbs, 0g fiber, 1g fat

Lettuce Wraps

1 tablespoon coconut oil	2 tablespoons Bragg Liquid Aminos
1 pound ground chicken or turkey breast	1 tablespoon rice vinegar
2 cloves garlic, minced (adjust to taste; we love garlic!)	2 teaspoons Thai chili paste
	Large iceberg or romaine lettuce leaves
½ teaspoon ground ginger	¼ cup chopped almonds
½ cup thinly sliced scallions	

Heat the oil in a large nonstick skillet over medium-high heat. Add the ground chicken or ground turkey, garlic, ginger, and scallions and cook thoroughly, breaking up the meat with a spatula as you go.

Whisk together the Bragg Liquid Aminos, vinegar, and chili paste in a small bowl. Pour the mixture over the meat and mix well. Dividing it evenly, top the lettuce leaves with the filling and then with chopped almonds. Roll up the leaves and enjoy!

SERVES 4

Per serving:
240 calories, 22g protein, 3g carbs, 1g fiber, 16g fat

Baked Mahi Mahi with Cilantro-Lime Sauce

1 tablespoon extra virgin olive oil	Juice of 1 lime
1 small bunch cilantro, finely chopped	1 pound mahi mahi fillets
2 cloves garlic, minced	Sea salt to taste

Preheat the oven to 400°F. Heat the olive oil in a small pan over medium-high heat. Add the cilantro, garlic, and lime juice and sauté for about 5 minutes, or until the cilantro is slightly wilted. Set aside. Place the fish in a glass baking dish and season with salt to taste. Spoon the oil mixture over the fish and bake, uncovered, for 15 minutes, or until the fish flakes easily.

SERVES 4

Per serving:
130 calories, 21g protein, 1g carbs, 0g fiber, 4.5g fat

CRUSHING CRAVINGS IN THE ELEL PHASE

Here are some of our favorite strategies for keeping HEC in check in the ELEL phase.

◎ **Fiber.** Adding a fiber supplement as a low-calorie "snack" between each of the three meals can have benefit in stopping hunger and cravings and improving fat loss. Ease into this gradually to make sure your digestive system can handle it without causing increased gas and bloating. For comparison with other brands, the one we use can be found here: metaboliceffect.com/product/fiber-complex.

◎ **Cocoa powder in water.** Slowly pour hot water over pure unsweetened baking cocoa in a mug (stirring to avoid clumping) for one of the most clinically effective tools we have ever seen at stopping cravings. This is especially useful for women during their menses. Because of its tryptamine content, cocoa can trigger migraines in some susceptible individuals, and it also can be too stimulating for some. For the vast majority, though, cocoa is a very gentle, extremely healthy means of crushing cravings that most people can even use at night with little impact on sleep.

⊚ **Craving cocoa.** After working with dieters for years, we developed this product that took the best natural craving reducer, cocoa, and spiked it with amino acids and viscous fibers to help eliminate hunger and cravings. You can find it on our site at: metaboliceffect.com/product/cravingcocoa.

⊚ **Lemon water.** Lemon is great for adding flavor to water and helping the digestive system. Add it in the morning, after meals, or whenever!

⊚ **Tea.** Black, green, and herbal teas (so long as they do not have added sweeteners) are great between meals and may even help some with a little extra fat-burning kick, due to their levels of the antioxidant epigallocatechin gallate (EGCG).

⊚ **Coffee.** The chlorogenic acid in coffee can increase levels of glucagon-like peptide 1 (GLP-1), a gut hormone that acts to turn off hunger. Adding cinnamon and cocoa can increase this effect (not to mention adding great taste to your coffee!). This effect is minimized, however, when adding any type of sweetener or milk, so drink coffee black. Be mindful of your individual reaction to coffee; while it can be a great way to suppress hunger in the short run, in some it can stimulate hunger and have blood sugar–changing effects.

⊚ **Water-based veggies like celery, peppers, and lettuce.** These are what we call water-based, negative-calorie foods. They do have calories, but they are called "negative-calorie foods" because it is believed the amount of energy it takes to digest these foods is probably close to the amount of calories they actually contain. Whether or not this is 100 percent true, you can eat bucketloads of this stuff and likely have very little negative caloric impact. If you are feeling true hunger in the gut, this stuff will certainly provide the bulk to shut it off.

⊚ **Branched-chain amino acids.** Branched-chain amino acids, abbreviated BCAAs, are essential amino acids. They are a special type of amino acid because they can easily be converted into glucose or the body's alternative fuel, ketones, if it is required. This means they are wonderful at stabilizing blood sugar and preventing low-sugar spells, or hypoglycemia. One of the key amino acids in this formula, leucine, also has effects on hunger in the brain. They also help raise levels of both the body's main relaxing brain chemical, GABA, and its major stimulating brain chemical, glutamate, thus having a nice balancing effect on brain chemistry. This multiaction effect on hunger suppression, brain chemistry, and blood sugar stabilization makes BCAA supplements a powerful ally to impact all parameters of HEC. Along with cocoa, BCAAs are one of the most effective things we have found clinically to stabilize HEC. They also have been shown to slow muscle loss caused by stress or a low-calorie diet. We

Eat Less, Exercise Less Protein Ratio Calculator

Numbers do weird things to our heads. Once we see numbers, we wrongly assume that everything is set in stone. Remember the idea of structured flexibility? Use this as a starting place and then tweak up and down as needed. Also, keep in mind this is an Eat Less, Exercise Less approach. Eating low calories while exercising like crazy is a very different thing from eating low calories while doing little exercise. Put your bias about how many calories you should or should not be eating aside and let your hunger-energy-cravings (HEC) reactions guide the adjustments. Your body knows best.

Though we want to wean you off of the calculator mentality, here's a tool to help you if you're numbers obsessed and you want to be specific about your intake.

Set your protein grams to your lean body mass.

Lean body mass (your muscle mass plus everything else in your body except fat) is calculated by subtracting your fat mass from your body weight. If Jane is 200 pounds and 30 percent body fat, her lean body mass would be calculated by multiplying 200×0.30, then subtracting that number from her weight.

$$200 \times 0.30 = 60$$
$$200 - 60 = 140$$

140 is the lean body mass. That is the grams of protein Jane will eat per day.

Calculate the total calories from protein.

There are 4 calories per gram of protein, so multiply your daily protein intake by 4.

$$140 \times 4 = 560$$

Jane will eat 560 calories of protein a day.

recommend taking 5 to 10 grams (5,000 to 10,000 milligrams) as a "snack" between the first and second meals during this stage. It is best to find a supplement that contains only the three BCAAs: leucine, isoleucine, and valine. Take note: These can be found in multiple forms at many health food stores, and many come heavily laced with artificial colorings and flavorings. As natural health care providers, we recommend avoiding these natural and artificial flavorings and sweeteners whenever possible, but we have to admit they do not seem to make any difference at all in the beneficial effects this supplement offers. And since straight BCAA powders are probably some of the worst-tasting amino-acid deliverers on the planet, we have learned to live with this

Calculate the daily calorie count.

Your diet should follow a carb-to-protein-to-fat ratio of 30:40:30. We know that Jane will be getting 560 calories from protein, so divide that amount by 0.40 to determine the daily calorie count.

560 ÷ 0.40 = 1,400

Jane's daily calorie count should be 1,400.

From the calorie count, calculate the carbs and fat.

Carbs and fat are each 30 percent of the diet, so Jane would multiply 1,400 by 0.30.

1,400 × 0.30 = 420

Jane's daily calories should include 420 calories of both carbs and fat.

1 gram of carbohydrates has 4 calories. To get Jane's daily carb intake in grams:

420 ÷ 4 = 105 grams of carbs

1 gram of fat has 9 calories. To get Jane's daily fat intake in grams:

420 ÷ 9 = 47 grams (really, 46.66 grams) of fat

So the breakdown of Jane's calories and macronutrients per day is:

1,400 calories
105 grams of carbs
140 grams of protein
47 grams of fat

We know, this is a lot of math. This is why we built an online calculator that will do the math for you. You can find it here: metaboliceffect.com/macro-calculator one downside. We recommend a brand called MRM BCAA+G Reload, which can be found online. While it does have some added ingredients and is not "pure" BCAAs, it's sweetened with natural ingredients, which we like.

◎ **Low-calorie powdered vegetable drinks.** These are basically the "fast food" version of the negative-calorie foods mentioned previously—when you add water, the powder gives you the same hydration, a small amount of fiber, and the phytonutrients that you would find in leafy greens and other vegetables. They're helpful on this plan because they can blunt hunger and provide some plant nutrition. Be very careful with these drinks and read the labels with care; many have high amounts of starch and sugar, making them harmful to your results. If you are going to incorporate these, choose ones with less than 10 grams of total carbs and 1 to 2 grams of fiber. The one we use in our clinic has a high prevalence of organic produce rather than grasses, fillers, and sugars: metaboliceffect.com/product/recovery-greens.

AVOIDING TRIGGER AND USING BUFFER FOODS

We all have metabolic differences. While we share overlapping metabolic similarities, we each have a unique insulin and blood sugar response to a given amount of food; different hunger, energy, and craving reactions to equal amounts of exercise; particular psychological sensitivities; and individual personal preferences. Because of this, we have reiterated that there is no one-size-fits-all approach to fitness and fat loss. You will constantly be playing diet detective as you work your way through our program. We'll give you suggestions along the way—things to look out for and assess—but the key to getting the shape you love and keeping it for life is being able to investigate your way into the perfect formula for you. It's a lifestyle we're helping you learn, not a diet, and our goal is to make it absent of cravings. You'll do so by achieving that state of metabolic balance we've mentioned.

Trigger foods and *buffer foods* can either get in your way or help. You'll need to be able to decipher them both, and in doing so, you will learn your own unique metabolic fat-loss formula.

Trigger Foods

A trigger food is one that causes undesirable effects after eating it and/or silently keeps you from achieving the diet and weight-loss results you're after. In other words, it *triggers* negative changes in your HEC, throwing it out of check and causing you to eat the wrong things. Trigger foods can also be foods that silently keep you from getting results due to hormonal changes, hidden sources of calories, or undesirable effects on the immune system.

Examples of Trigger Foods

◎ **Artificial sweeteners** have zero calories, but they can easily disrupt biochemistry. These sweeteners may trigger what is known as the cephalic phase insulin response. This is a mechanism by which the sweet taste acts neurologically through the tongue (called the neurolingual connection) to induce insulin secretion by the pancreas. In other words, the body tastes something sweet, so it expects to find sugar in the bloodstream soon after it gets a taste. As a result, it releases insulin. But when the sugar does not come, the released insulin can end up lowering blood sugar instead. That may then cause the brain to increase hunger and cravings, as it perceives a low blood sugar threat. Some people who consume these end up with insatiable hunger and cravings. Some, however, see no effect and may even benefit from using artificial sweeteners. Our bias is to avoid them, of course, but an honest review of the literature suggests that much of the negative media hype about these things is mostly hype. We prefer you avoid them to err on the side of caution, but if you must use them, you should be aware of what impact they may have. Understanding these individual reactions is key. Your job is to play detective to assess if it is an issue for you.

◎ **Natural no-calorie sweeteners** can have the same effects as artificial sweeteners. If you are going to use low-cal and no-cal sweeteners, use natural compounds like stevia and the natural sugar alcohols xylitol and erythritol. We do advise you to proceed with caution, though, since they can still be triggers for cravings in some people.

◎ **Dairy and gluten** can interrupt metabolism through immune mechanisms. This is quickly becoming one of the fastest-growing areas of research in endocrinology and immunology. We now know that many more people than we ever thought are reacting to gluten in subtle ways that may be negatively impacting metabolic function. So, there is much truth to the idea that gluten can pose an issue for some. Of course, in our integrative medicine clinic we deal with this every single day, but we think it is irresponsible for many in the natural medicine world to sound alarms that make it seem like gluten is the next black plague. Again, we now know that things like gluten sensitivities and immune reactions to other foods can and do impact the immune and hormonal metabolism, but to assume this is the case in all or most people simply is not warranted. Later on we will teach you how to do some more detective work to determine if you may be impacted. The good news is that following our simple 3-2-1 protocol and using hypoallergenic shakes virtually eliminates both dairy and gluten from the diet effortlessly.

◎ **Fruits, sugar-free products, nuts and nut butters, and alcohol** can all trigger compensatory eating reactions that lead to eating too much food and/ or the wrong types of food later. They also can simply have more or less of a fat-storing effect in certain people. Nuts are usually inefficiently digested, so their fat can pass through the digestive system and not be absorbed. People with more efficient digestion may extract more of the fat from nuts than others. That is just one example of how these foods can help some and hurt others.

◎ **The combination of fat, starch, sugar, and salt** can be a trigger, too. Highly palatable foods such as these make us eat more at the present meal and cause brain changes that make us crave more of those foods later. This is why cheat meals can be such a slippery slope and go from a cheat meal to a cheat month. This is a very hot area of research. And we have come to see this as a highly important factor in food cravings and overeating. To avoid this combination, we suggest you isolate your macronutrients whenever possible, choosing foods that do not combine fats, sugars, starches, and salt to avoid the druglike craving effect these foods may have in susceptible people.

◎ **Foods with high-flavor profiles** can also be triggers, which means a heads-up for the foodies reading. The more variety in flavor, the more we eat and the more we crave. We realize it is not fun and it might piss you off a bit, but the truth of the matter is that the simplest diet may actually be the least likely to cause cravings.

◎ **A limited-variety diet** can also be a trigger for some. Some research suggests that when the food choices are too limited, that can cause exaggerated responses when more food options are presented. We realize this point seems to contradict the previous point. Nutrition information often seems this way. The take-away is to vary your food choices, but keep the flavor profiles and food combinations minimized. We don't want to make you neurotic, but we do want you to understand that food combinations impact us in ways that are not as apparent as the caloric count of a meal. *What* you eat can impact *how much* you eat, and also impact what and how much you eat at your next meal. So, basically, the ideal diet is one with a variety of food groups, but without too many flavor profiles.

Buffer Foods

If you're struggling to stay on track during the week, then the buffer foods, unlike the trigger foods, may work for you, not against you. Used periodically during the week, buffer foods have the ability to balance your metabolism. They vary more broadly compared to trigger foods and could be something that is merely psychologically pleasing. For example, if you have two small squares of dark chocolate in the afternoon when you're craving candy, you might not go to the candy machine at work for an entire bag of M&M's or you might avoid ordering a large pepperoni pizza later that night. Simply put: Buffer foods can keep you sane. They buffer the negative impact of fluctuations in hunger, energy, and cravings, making them a great tool for you to use to manage this lifestyle and, ultimately, body change.

Now, keep in mind: This isn't an open invitation to eat platefuls of buffer foods, but you'll see the value in them in controlling urges and preventing you from making bigger mistakes later. To a large extent, the use of buffer foods is a spin on the old adage of "everything in moderation." But if you eat buffer foods in huge amounts, they can become trigger foods, so tread lightly. And remember that a trigger food for one person might be a buffer food for another person. One useful guideline for finding out if a food is a buffer food is to ask yourself, "Can I control my intake of this food?" A food that you can't stop eating is not a buffer food, but a food you can eat a small amount of and feel satisfied by is. There is no black and white here. We hope you're getting used to that idea, because it is the real way this game of metabolic detective works.

Examples of Buffer Foods

- Sparkling water
- Nut butters
- Salt
- Dark chocolate or cocoa
- Sugar-free products
- Nuts and seeds

- High-fat foods like avocado and sour cream
- Cheese
- Salty, fatty meats like bacon and hot dogs
- A cocktail or glass of wine

AN UNTRADITIONAL CALORIE DEFICIT

This 3-2-1 phase is indeed creating a calorie deficit, but not traditionally, the way you might think. We're doing it by also creating metabolic balance instead of having you eat less and exercise more. In the Eat Less, Exercise Less (ELEL) phase, we've got you doing what our grandparents did, not running around like crazy exercising, but staying lean because they kept the eating in check. It will yield a lean physique by essentially starving that stubborn fat. This plan takes care to provide adequate protein to help control hunger and maintain muscle. It's not just that we're trying to cut the calories down here; we're also trying to clear out the metabolic smoke so people can clearly see the signals their metabolism is sending. The reason we suggest you do this phase for 2 weeks is because that's about how long it takes for the metabolism to respond and adjust to this new approach. Every time you change your eating, it takes from several days to a couple of weeks to adjust to it, in terms of both eating habits and metabolic output. If you're really doing well and your metabolism is really flexible, you'll start seeing a difference within 4 to 7 days. Two weeks gives you enough time to adequately measure the impact, and this is about the time it takes for the metabolism to adapt as well. In addition to eating and exercising appropriately, there are two more key tools to success in this phase: sleep and mindfulness.

Get Your Sleep

We've given you an eating plan and exercise guidelines, but there is another critical ingredient to this reshaping of your body and breaking down of those trouble spots: sleep. You need 7 to 9 hours of it, and that might be the most significant component of this entire weight-loss puzzle. It is the hormonal reset button. It will impact how much and what you eat the next day. People who don't get adequate sleep have more cravings, are hungrier, have less motivation to work out, and have more depression and anxiety. As a result, they gain weight.

Be Mindful

The other key factor in all of this is being mindful. It's a theme we like to follow in general, especially with the dinner meal in the 3-2-1 phase. Be mindful and enjoy your meal. Also, no matter how busy your life is, don't wait around for some "better" time to start doing this. Don't wait until life is calm or an event is over, because you need to live your life. Jump in.

THE EXERCISE LESS APPROACH

Let's review now how the Exercise Less portion of this phase works. If you're going to be eating less, you certainly shouldn't exercise more (contrary to what conventional diets tell you!). If you exercise more while eating less, you will enter dieting mode and cause metabolic compensation and disrupted HEC. If you're currently sedentary, this phase will obviously mean you're moving *more* than you're used to, but it's not going to be so much exercise that it disrupts your HEC. It will be enough to work with your diet and blast fat.

MOVING VERSUS EXERCISE

There is a slight difference between moving and exercising. We define "movement" as a form of transportation or activities of daily living, and it has been a necessity for all of human history. "Exercise" as we think of it is a modern-day construct that was not engaged in by the population outside of athletes until the late 1960s and 1970s. Understanding this distinction between movement and exercise will help you understand how each impacts stress and HEC. In general, movement is stress relieving and has a minimal impact on HEC. Exercise, on the other hand, can quickly become a stress on the body, especially if it is combined with less food intake, as traditional Eat Less, Exercise More approaches prescribe.

So while this stage is an Eat Less, Exercise Less approach, it is also an eat less, move regularly approach. Moving is critical to this phase. It may surprise you to know that movement is far more beneficial to weight loss and health than exercise. Research shows those who move all day but do no exercise fare better than those who sit all day but do exercise for 30 to 60 minutes. We encourage you to move as often as you can, always remaining aware of the difference between movement and exercise.

Suggested Movements in the ELEL Phase

◎ Slow, leisurely walking for 1 to 2 hours (about 5,000–10,000 steps)

◎ Standing instead of sitting whenever possible

◎ Taking the stairs instead of the elevator

◎ Fidgeting while you sit

◎ Taking every opportunity to move in the same way you would if you lived in a more natural setting

We encourage you to use an activity tracker to gain valuable feedback on each day's movement. Just remember to measure movement, not exercise, with it. We love the Fitbit; you can get one on their site (bit.ly/MEfitbit).

EXERCISE SMART

Most people assume exercise is the best way to burn fat. Put simply, it's not. Your diet is what unlocks your ability to burn fat. Imagine a fat cell as a house stuffed with fat. You can run around the house checking all the doors like crazy, but if the doors are locked, the fat is never coming out. This is analogous to using exercise to try to burn fat—it is futile without a proper diet, since it's the diet that unlocks and opens the doors. Once your diet is balanced, however, adding exercise can speed the release of fat.

Exercise can create another problem, which is often called the "halo effect." This occurs when one healthy action (say, spending an hour on the treadmill) casts a positive "halo" over a less healthy thing and then gives psychological license to overindulge. When some people exercise, they often overestimate how many calories they've burned, and therefore how many calories they're "allowed" to consume because of it. You can spend an entire hour on a treadmill just to wipe out all progress in the 90 seconds it takes you to eat half a bagel. The halo effect is also a result of falling into the calorie trap and calculator game. You now know this is not the way the metabolism works.

Exercise and Your HEC

Exercise also impacts HEC, and the type you do can impact how much you eat and what you choose to eat later. Exercise is neither healthy nor weight-loss friendly if it causes you to crave and eat too much of the wrong foods later. Long hours spent running or jogging can prompt those kinds of hunger and craving reactions. For a lot of people, running or jogging is alluring because it "feels" like you're working toward weight loss—but if you're constantly fighting your hunger and cravings after a long run, you are fighting a losing battle.

Don't look at exercise as just calorie burning. Some people may think the longer they can go, the more calories they will burn, and the better off they will be. We want you to understand that exercise is not just about calories. It's about hormones too. How exercise impacts your hormonal chemistry during a workout will affect hunger, energy, and cravings after the workout.

Exercise That Increases Hunger and Cravings

Exercise that is longer and more intense will usually increase hunger and cravings shortly after the workout is complete. People who are overweight and obese often have metabolic issues that make them suffer more cravings and hunger than lean people, making them especially susceptible to this. Examples of exercise that might increase your hunger and cravings are:

- Running
- Biking
- Jogging
- Power walking

This certainly is not true for all people, but for many it is. Part of your detective work is figuring out which exercise works best for you. So observe closely: If you are negatively impacted by exercise in this way, you may want to limit moderate or intense exercise sessions to less than an hour.

Exercise that is shorter and more intense often has an appetite-suppressing effect in the hours after the workout and may even make you feel nauseated immediately afterward, but it too can increase hunger and cravings later. Examples include:

- Interval training
- Intense weight training
- Metabolic-conditioning workouts
- Sprint training

This type of exercise causes a short-term delay in hunger and then an uptick in hunger and cravings later. To combat the cravings and hunger that follow these types of exercises, eat healthy, HEC-stabilizing foods like a quick protein recovery shake or a large salad with chicken during this brief time when cravings for palatable foods are low. This should keep those cravings from popping up later.

Exercise That Decreases Hunger and Cravings

If you are going to exercise for a long period of time, slow, relaxing movement is really your best choice, and a priority in this phase. Very-low-intensity exercise tends to have little impact on hunger and cravings, and may actually decrease cravings since it has such a nice impact on lowering stress hormones like cortisol. Examples of these kinds of exercise include:

- Relaxing and restorative yoga (such as Anusara, hatha, Kripalu, yin, or Taoist)
- Tai chi
- Slow, leisurely walking

Walking, which really qualifies more as movement than exercise, should be a dominant form of activity in your life, especially in the Eat Less, Exercise Less phase of restoring metabolic function and starving the fat. You really can't do too much slow, relaxing walking. Notice here we use the terms *slow* and *relaxing*? Power walking is not the same as leisure walking. Leisurely walking is what is most beneficial in lowering cortisol secretion, while power walking may raise it.

You should notice right away that when you start looking at exercise as both hormonal and caloric, it changes your outlook. Going for a long run that burns 500 calories but then results in having a dinner in which you eat an extra 1,000 calories is a worse choice than going for a slow walk that only burns 100 calories, but leads to eating 300 calories less than you normally would.

THE 3-2-1 EXERCISE PLAN

◎ 3 or more rest and recovery activities per week (you can't do too many)

◎ 2 traditional weight-training workouts per week

◎ 1 hour or more of slow, leisurely walking on all or most days (you can't do too much of this)

3 Rest and Recovery Sessions

You can do any of a number of cortisol-lowering activities. Take a hot Epsom salts bath, get a massage, have sex (orgasms are a fantastic de-stressor!), do a restorative yoga class, play with your pet, do tai chi, or just have a nap. These may not sound like critical components to losing weight, but trust us, they are. These activities retrain the nervous system to be able to be in rest, recovery, and repair mode. Your damaged metabolism desperately needs this time. This speaks to the difference between sympathetic (fight or flight) versus parasympathetic (rest and digest) physiology. The bottom line: Most of us are extremely overstressed. We

Too Much Screen Time Spells Trouble

Watching TV and using the computer may seem relaxing, and for the first 15 minutes or so, they might be. But if you have ever sat in front of a TV all day, you know that rarely does it leave you rested and restored. This peculiar phenomenon in which an activity first makes you feel relaxed, but then causes fatigue or lethargy, is referred to by psychology researchers as "psychic entropy." This is a term that speaks to the slow loss of mental energy that accompanies these behaviors. So, we are not saying here that you should not watch TV; we are saying that TV can be a slippery slope for rest and relaxation. A small amount is probably fine, but too much can thwart your success. Whenever possible, we suggest you seek relaxation activities that do *not* include TV or computer time. One notable exception to this rule may be funny shows and movies. Laughter is a wonderful way to lower stress hormones.

like to say that you can eat your way to obesity, or you can stress yourself there. These rest and recovery activities help alleviate some of your stress.

2 Exercise Sessions

These constitute two traditional weight-training sessions per week. By "traditional," we mean standard weight training—full-body workouts. Popular metabolic-conditioning workouts (like our Metabolic Effect workouts or CrossFit workouts) are often seen as acceptable replacements for traditional weight training, but they really aren't, since they do not do a great job of overloading muscles in a way that stimulates muscle growth or maintenance. In other words, these workouts are great for helping burn fat when the diet is right, but they don't efficiently help maintain and/or gain muscle.

In the 3-2-1 workout, you'll do four exercises: shoulder presses, squats, bent-over rows, and pushups. Do 4 or 5 sets of 8 to 12 reps for each exercise, using a weight heavy enough that it makes the last reps almost impossible to lift with proper form. Be sure to take 1- to 3-minute rests between sets. This rest is very beneficial to retraining proper sympathetic and parasympathetic balance. You don't want to overtax the body and lose muscle mass, and fast-paced metabolic conditioning can sometimes overtax the system. If you absolutely can't give up your fast-paced exercise regimen and must do it instead, then we suggest doing it no more than twice a week during this stage. The goal with this traditional weight training is to tax the body with heavy weights and then allow it to recover before repeating.

Do 4 or 5 sets of each of these four exercises, keeping in mind:

◎ Choose a weight heavy enough that it is very difficult to complete 10 reps in each set.

◎ If you can do more than 12 reps, then increase the weight.

◎ If you can't get at least 8 reps, then reduce the weight.

Your ELEL Equipment

◎ Two dumbbells. Choose a weight heavy enough that you can complete only 10 reps in each set.

◎ Scale

◎ Tape measure

◎ Inclined adjustable bench (recommended, but not mandatory)

THE 3-2-1 WORKOUT

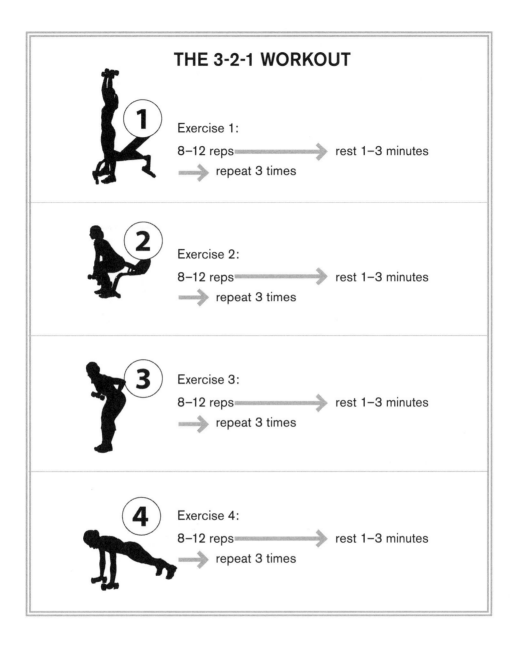

(1) Exercise 1:

8–12 reps ➤ rest 1–3 minutes

➤ repeat 3 times

(2) Exercise 2:

8–12 reps ➤ rest 1–3 minutes

➤ repeat 3 times

(3) Exercise 3:

8–12 reps ➤ rest 1–3 minutes

➤ repeat 3 times

(4) Exercise 4:

8–12 reps ➤ rest 1–3 minutes

➤ repeat 3 times

If you are using dumbbells, a quick way to figure out your 10-rep max is to find a weight you can lift with good form no more than three times and then cut that number in half.

(1) SHOULDER PRESS

Stand with your feet together and a slight bend in your knees. Hold two dumbbells at shoulder height with your palms facing your shoulders. Keep your chest up and your head and neck straight while looking straight in front of you. Now press the weights straight up toward the ceiling until your elbows are almost locked and your palms face each other. Lower the weights slowly, keeping them under control, until they are back to shoulder height. Repeat until you've completed as many as you can while still maintaining good form, for a total of 8 to 12 times.

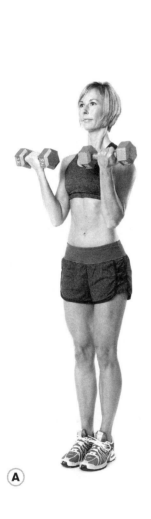

(A)

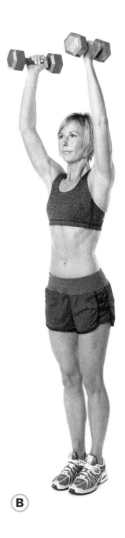

(B)

② SQUAT

Stand with the dumbbells hanging at arm's length at your sides or a barbell across your back at the shoulders. Keep your chest and head up. Bending at your hips and knees, squat downward and backward as if you're going to sit in a chair. Lower yourself until your thighs are parallel with the floor or even lower at your hips. Now push hard through your heels to stand back up. Repeat to complete 8 to 12 reps. Those who need a bit more of a strength challenge may want to do the Bulgarian Split Squat instead.

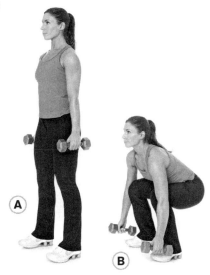

BULGARIAN SPLIT SQUAT:

With your arms hanging at your sides without dumbbells, move into the lunge position, with your front foot flat on the floor beneath your torso and the toes of your back foot resting on a bench or chair behind you. Keep your chest high, your tummy tight, and your neck straight while you look straight ahead. Your front foot should be pointing straight ahead. Now drop the back knee down to the floor. This will cause the front knee to bend. Drop down until the thigh of the forward leg is parallel to the floor. Be sure to keep your head and chest up. Push hard down through the heel of the front foot and raise yourself back up. Repeat for 8 to 12 total. If this is too easy and you can do more than 12 reps, then add dumbbells to the exercise. After completing 8 to 12 reps on one leg, switch and do 8 to 12 reps on the other leg.

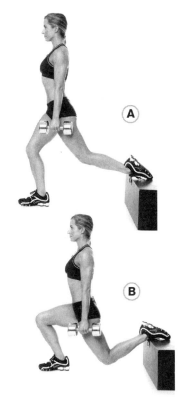

③ BENT-OVER ROW

Holding a dumbbell in each hand at your sides with your arms straight, bend your knees slightly and push your butt back so you are slightly leaning over your legs. Keep your lower back flat so you aren't arching your torso too far back or bending it too far forward. Your torso should be at a 45-degree angle to the floor. Let the dumbbells hang straight down, perpendicular to the floor, just to the outside and slightly in front of your knees. Keep your weight in your legs. Now pull the weights up by pulling your elbows back and up toward the ceiling. This should cause your shoulder blades to pinch together and the weights should end up positioned alongside your torso, between your underarms and belly button. Return the weights to the straight-arm position and repeat for a total of 8 to 12 times. The proper form for this exercise can be very difficult for some beginners to achieve. If you feel too much stress in your lower back, sit in a chair, lean over your legs, and do the movement from there. If you have access to a gym, you may choose to use the back row machine. Advanced weight lifters will likely choose to use a barbell instead of dumbbells for this exercise in order to increase the weight.

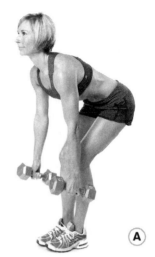

(A)

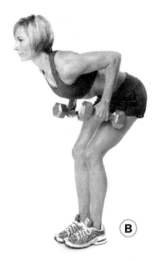

(B)

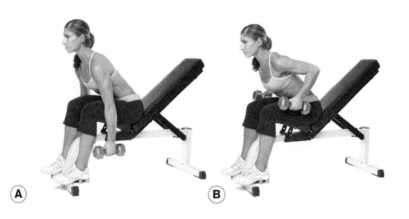

(A)   (B)

(4) PUSHUP

Start in a plank position with your hands shoulder-width apart and in line with your chest. Your neck should be straight, with your eyes looking straight down at the floor. Keep your feet together and balance on your toes; if you can't do toe pushups, drop to your knees, keeping them close together. Keep your core tight by imagining a string is pulling your belly button back to your spine. Now lower yourself slowly to the floor until your chest touches it. Keep your hands rotated slightly outward so your elbows are closer to your torso rather than flaring out to the sides. Now push hard with your chest and arms to push yourself back to the up position. Repeat to complete 8 to 12 pushups. If you are a more advanced weight lifter and pushups are too easy for you, feel free to sub in the Decline Pushup or a Heavy Bench Press here.

DECLINE PUSHUP:

Put your feet on a chair or bench instead of the floor. This increases the tension and how much weight the chest muscles must lift.

HEAVY BENCH PRESS:

A heavy bench press will also load more weight onto the chest; use heavier dumbbells or even a barbell, which you can load more weight on.

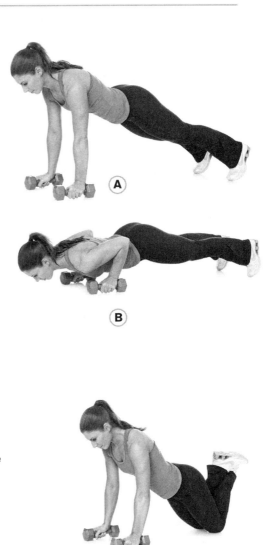

1- to 2-Hour Walking Sessions

These slow, leisurely walks should be done on all or most days of the week, and they are the most critical aspect of the ELEL phase. Leisure walking is incredibly healing to the metabolism: It doesn't impact your hunger and cravings the way high-intensity cardio can, and it keeps your muscle tissue and liver very sensitive to the hormone insulin. Leisure walking is one of the few activities that lower cortisol levels and balance the nervous system. This means it helps the body deal with stress in a healthy and productive manner. You really cannot do too much walking, and we encourage you to do as much as you like. Make sure you're moving at a pace equivalent to walking a dog. It's not power walking. You should be able to carry on a conversation and not be out of breath.

The Exercise Obsessed

We know there will be those of you reading this who will say that you love exercise so much that this just won't be enough for you. You think you'll go crazy if you're not moving. But if you want the best results, during these 2 weeks, try to stick to this 3-2-1 protocol. If you refuse to follow our advice and insist upon exercising more than is outlined here, there are a couple of things to keep in mind.

1. It really is not ideal and could hurt your results.

2. If you must exercise more, then you must adjust your food intake so you are not in an Eat Less, Exercise More state. Do not exceed the following guidelines.

For the workout obsessed, the 3-2-1 guide will keep excess exercise in check.

◎ "3" means no more than three intense or long-duration exercise sessions per week. If you really must do CrossFit or marathon running or something similarly intense, then try to limit it to 3 times per week. We warn you, though: You're not going to get the best results from this protocol because you'll be tipping into the Eat Less, Exercise More world.

◎ "2" means at least 2 rest and relaxation activities.

◎ "1" means keep up the walking. It is still great for you and the relaxing qualities may help offset some of the stress from the excess exercise.

The Goldilocks Zone: Hunger

The ability to fill up fast from a meal and stay satisfied for a long period of time is a direct reflection of your brain's sensitivity to insulin and leptin. Both hormones control hunger, and the brain has to be able to "hear" their signals, or, in science-speak, remain "sensitive" to them.

Think of hormone levels like Goldilocks. They can't be too low or too high, instead needing to be *just right*. Leptin and insulin are two of the most critical hormones in this regard.

Leptin comes from your fat cells. When your fat cells grow, leptin is released. Leptin then goes up to the brain and tells it, "Hey, brain, we have enough fat on our body. So please stop eating so much. Be more full and satisfied." Leptin will also go to the thyroid and adrenal glands to stimulate an increase in metabolism.

But if too much leptin is produced, your body stops listening to it. You can become leptin and insulin resistant. If too little leptin or insulin is produced, you will be hungry all the time. But have too much, and you create the same issue. You will be hungry all the time and your metabolism will slow down. This is why dietary extremes of low carbs and low calories almost always backfire.

If you pay close attention to your hunger, you will learn to know whether your leptin and insulin are balanced appropriately for you.

Cravings

The same goes for cravings; they can act as biofeedback on your stress hormones, such as cortisol. Stress impacts the brain by turning down the goal centers while ramping up the reward centers. Cortisol is involved in this. Ghrelin, a hunger hormone released from the stomach, also impacts cravings.

If you are overweight or obese and you're always hungry and having cravings, you might be insulin and leptin resistant, and you are likely producing high levels of stress hormones. This is why focusing on HEC is so critical. If the 3-2-1 approach is not working, adjust to the 5-4-1 (see page 66). You'll eat every 2 to 4 hours, instead of every 4 to 6 hours. In a sense, we've got you counting your hormones instead of your calories, which will in turn help you balance your metabolism.

THE LOSE WEIGHT HERE RECAP

◎ Follow the ELEL phase for 2 weeks.

◎ Follow a 3-2-1 eating plan (3 meals a day; 2 meals are protein-based and sugar- and starch-free; 1 meal is a regular 3-2-1 meal).

◎ Regular meals adhere to 3-2-1 proportions on the plate: 3 parts vegetables, 2 parts protein, 1 part starch.

◎ Exercise less to allow your body to focus on starving the fat.

◎ Follow the simple 3-2-1 exercise plan: 3 or more rest and recovery activities per week, 2 traditional weight-training workouts per week, and 1 to 2 hours (about 5,000 to 10,000 steps) of slow, leisurely walking on all or most days.

Remember: 3-2-1 for both food and exercise for 2 weeks. Eat Less, Exercise Less. Assess, investigate, and modify as needed to make this phase really work for you.

CHAPTER 6

FEED THE LEAN PHASE:

Eat More,
Exercise More

The starve-the-fat stage was about stripping clay from the sculpture. We were giving the metabolism a much-needed break from dieting and repairing the metabolic damage caused by the dieting lifestyle. The 3-2-1 phase was mostly about depriving your fat cells and forcing them to let go of the fat instead of holding on to it.

This second phase is about shaping the body's precise contours. It is about what we call "feeding the lean." Imagine a sculptor carving a figure's fine details and creating edges and curves. That's what you will be doing during this phase. You will continue burning fat, but you will shift your focus more to toning your muscles.

In this phase, you will work with the Law of Metabolic Compensation by cycling the diet in a way that stops metabolic compensation and maximizes your potential to both burn fat and tone muscle. The Eat More, Exercise More phase will have you doing short, intense exercise sessions lasting 20 minutes on 6 days a week in addition to a continued focus on lots of slow, leisurely walking. You will also ramp up your fat and/or starch intake for muscle recovery, repair, and regeneration.

"Cycling" means that you will switch back and forth between the Eat More, Exercise More (EMEM) approach and the Eat Less, Exercise Less (ELEL) approach you've been doing for the past 2 weeks. You'll follow each cycle for a 2-week period, alternating back and forth until you reach your goal.

Once you complete the EMEM cycle, you will switch back to the ELEL approach for 2 weeks. The norm will become alternating between these two approaches every 2 weeks, monitoring your results as you go, for as long as it takes for you to reach your goal size, weight, and shape. It typically takes 2 to 3 months if you have less than 30 pounds to lose and 3 to 12 months if you have more.

In this phase, your results are measured by the number of pounds shed but, more importantly, by the number of inches lost. Plan on losing between 1 and 4 inches in your stubborn-fat areas while dropping between 2 and 8 pounds—and up to 2 percent of your body fat.

EMEM AT A GLANCE

The 4-2-2 Eating Plan

What does your 4-2-2 eating day look like?

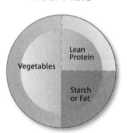

The 4-2-2 Meal Plate

◎ 4 meals per day

◎ 2 of those meals are protein shakes or protein and vegetable based.

◎ 2 of those meals are regular meals containing starch and are best consumed after you've done your workout.

◎ Enjoy up to two reward or cheat meals each week if your results and response to cheat meals indicate you can; for example, they help you keep your hunger-energy-cravings (HEC) in check and get good fat-loss results—and don't lead to a cheat week.

The two regular meals can be thought of in terms of 4-2-2 proportions on the plate: 4 parts vegetables, 2 parts protein, and 2 parts starch and/or fat. Protein sources should weigh about 8 ounces.

The 4-2-2 Exercise Plan

You will also follow a 4-2-2 exercise plan. These numbers denote weekly goals, not daily goals like in the eating plan.

What does a snapshot of your 4-2-2 exercise week look like?

◎ 4 metabolic chain workouts per week (20 minutes each)

◎ 2 rest-based interval training (RBIT) sessions per week (20 minutes each)

◎ 2 hours or more (about 10,000 to 20,000 steps) of leisurely walking on as many days as possible

The chains and the interval work will use two tools: rest-based training and metabolic conditioning, specifically our brand of conditioning called Metabolic Physique Conditioning.

NOTE: If you are a runner, you may replace some of the leisurely walking with running. Just remember, this can easily be overdone and throw HEC out of check. So make sure it works for you. If it does, feel free to add two or three sessions during the week in place of the walking.

The 4-2-2 Week

A sample week on this plan might look like this.

DAY	MEAL 1	MEAL 2	MEAL 3	MEAL 4	EXERCISE	WALK
Monday	Vegetable egg frittata, small bowl of berries	Protein smoothie (20 to 40 grams of protein powder in unsweetened almond, coconut, or low-fat [1% or 2%] cow's milk or water) or protein snack	Spinach-chicken wrap	2 cups broccoli, 8 ounces grilled halibut, 1 sweet potato, pat of butter	Metabolic chain session: burpee chain for 20 minutes	Accumulate about 10,000–20,000 steps
Tuesday	1 to 2 cups full-fat Greek yogurt, ½ cup strawberries, ½ cup bananas, or a combination of the two	Protein smoothie made with a banana	Large Caesar salad with salmon	Vegetable chicken stir-fry	Rest-based interval training	

DAY	MEAL 1	MEAL 2	MEAL 3	MEAL 4	EXERCISE	WALK
Wednesday	Protein pancakes (almond flour, oats, egg whites)	Protein smoothie made with a banana	Burrito bowl with extra chicken, veggies, and salsa (no rice, beans, or starch)	Spaghetti squash with tomato sauce, grilled chicken	Metabolic chain session: leg chain for 20 minutes	2 hours of leisurely walking (about 10,000–20,000 steps)
Thursday	Protein smoothie or protein- and vegetable-based snack	Protein smoothie or protein- and vegetable-based snack	Chicken and vegetable teriyaki, ½ cup cooked white rice	Mixed vegetables, salmon, sweet potato	Rest-based interval training	
Friday	Oatmeal mixed with 20 grams protein powder	Protein smoothie made with a banana	Large salad with grilled chicken	New York strip steak, broccoli, glass of red wine	Metabolic chain session: incline chain for 20 minutes	2 hours of leisurely walking (about 10,000–20,000 steps)
Saturday	Scrambled eggs, Canadian bacon, berries	Protein smoothie or protein- and vegetable-based snack	Protein smoothie made with a banana	Free meal	Metabolic chain session: burpee chain for 20 minutes	2 hours of leisurely walking (about 10,000–20,000 steps)
Sunday	Protein pancakes (almond flour, oats, egg whites)	Protein smoothie or protein- and vegetable-based snack	1 cup beanless, starchless chili	Free meal		

THE EAT MORE APPROACH

The one significant difference you'll likely notice most in this phase is the added starch. Remember what we have been saying: A low-carb, healthy meal is neither low carb nor healthy if it makes you eat worse foods later. Starches are not the enemy, and they just may be the very thing that keeps your HEC in check, allowing you to finally turn dieting into a lifestyle. They also have special application during this Eat More, Exercise More, or "feed the lean," part of the program: They help tone muscle and allow you to lower stress hormone levels. Opt for the higher fiber and "wetter" versions of these foods (like brown rice and potatoes with the skin on). Try not to add fat (such as olive oil or butter) to these foods—try seasoning with a little salt and pepper instead.

Putting Your Meals Together

In the EMEM approach, like in ELEL, you can mix and match to suit your tastes. Here, though, are some general guidelines.

- ◎ Your plate should be comprised of 4 parts veggies, 2 parts protein, and 2 parts starches or fats (only the two meals that include starch).
- ◎ Stick with lean protein sources.
- ◎ Add fat separately.
- ◎ Eat veggies and proteins before starches.
- ◎ If you aren't satiated after your meal, you may need more protein.

Tips on Protein

Part of the reason we want you to focus on lean proteins instead of fatty ones is because it's easier to play metabolic detective when these types of macronutrients are kept separate. If fat is included with your protein, you aren't really able to identify which one is controlling your HEC. By getting protein and fat, however, from different sources, you can add and subtract fat more easily (for example by adding a few wedges of avocado, olives, or oil). And, therefore, you can more easily determine how protein and fat are individually impacting your HEC, allowing you to track the results. So, your diet should not be low fat or high fat—it should be *your* fat—whatever amount it is that balances HEC, helps you burn fat, and keeps you healthy and vital. It's really about developing the ability to know how fat is affecting you.

We want you to understand the differences between protein foods, fat-based foods, and foods that are mostly starch. For example, beans are *not* considered a protein on this plan—even though they have some protein in them, they're more starch than anything else. Nuts are also not considered protein sources; they're mostly fat. Proteins, essentially, are foods that are more protein than anything else. (The same goes for fat- and starch-rich foods.) Looking at food this way allows you to become an expert at playing metabolic detective with your food, since you can adjust individual macronutrient intake for pinpointed responses.

Fat-Loss-Food Cheat Sheet

Protein: Lean versus Fatty

Lean proteins: chicken, turkey, wild fowl, game meats, most fish, bison, lean ground beef, shellfish, and lean cuts of pork

Fatty meats: lamb, fatty cuts of beef, fatty cuts of pork, and fatty fish like salmon

Veggies: Nonstarchy versus Starchy

Nonstarchy high-fiber veggies: kale, collards, Brussels sprouts, broccoli, cabbage, cauliflower, spinach, lettuce, salad greens, tomato, jicama, asparagus, green beans, cucumber, celery, bell peppers, carrot, radish, zucchini, squashes, and pumpkin

Starchy low-fiber veggies: potatoes, corn, peas, and sweet potatoes

Fruits: High Water versus Low Water versus High Sugar

High water, low sugar: berries, apples, pears, and citrus fruits

High water, higher sugar: bananas, melons, cherries, pineapples, mango, and kiwifruit

Low water: raisins, dried cranberries, apricots, prunes, and other dried fruits

Starches: Wet versus Dry

Wet starches: potatoes, corn, peas, sweet potatoes, rice, quinoa, oats, cream of rice, and beans and legumes

Dry starches: pastas, breads, crackers, pretzels, chips, rice cakes, and cereals

Fats

Avocado, olives and olive oil, coconut oil, butter and ghee, vegetable oils, nuts and seeds, and peanuts

As you can see from this chart, fat-loss foods rich in protein, fiber, and water (the green foods) are best at stabilizing HEC and contain the fewest calories. They tend to fill us up quickly, making us less likely to eat more of the wrong foods later. They can be eaten in unlimited quantities by most people, because they are so satiating and so low in calories.

The yellow foods list includes foods that have a varied impact from person to person. For some, these foods balance HEC and aid fat loss. For others, the very same foods will not stabilize HEC and may lead to fat gain. It is with these foods that people will have to do most of their detective work.

Foods listed as red foods have a negative impact on hunger-energy-cravings (HEC), either decreasing fullness at the meal or making overeating at that meal or future meals more likely. These foods have the most potential to cause fat gain. Pastas, cereals, and breads are examples. These foods

How Foods Affect HEC and Fat Storage

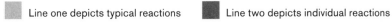

Line one depicts typical reactions   Line two depicts individual reactions

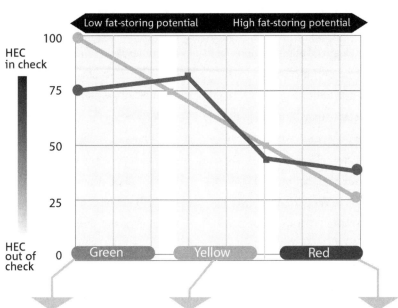

Green (eat unlimited)	Yellow (eat to tolerance)	Red (eat rarely if ever)
Protein/Veg: chicken, turkey, wild fowl, game meats, most fish, bison, lean ground beef, shellfish, lean cuts of pork, egg whites, and protein powders	**Fatty meats:** lamb, fatty cuts of beef, fatty cuts of pork, fatty fish like salmon	**Dry starches:** pasta, bread, crackers, pretzels, chips, rice cakes, cereals
	Vegetable fats: avocado, olives, olive oil, coconut oil, vegetable oils, nuts and seeds, peanuts	**Junk foods:** cookies, cakes, candy, sweets, soda, etc.
Nonstarchy high-fiber veggies: kale, collards, Brussels sprouts, broccoli, cabbage, cauliflower, spinach, lettuce, salad greens, tomato, jicama, asparagus, green beans, cucumber, celery, peppers, carrots, radish, zucchini, squashes, pumpkin	**Lower-fiber, high-sugar fruits:** banana, melons, cherries, pineapples, mango, kiwi	
	Starchy low-fiber veggies: potatoes, corn, peas, sweet potatoes	
High-water, low-sugar fruits: berries, apples, pears, citrus fruits	**Wet starches:** potatoes, corn, peas, sweet potatoes, rice, quinoa, oats, cream of rice, beans and legumes	
	Dairy foods: milk, yogurt, butter, cheese	
	Whole eggs	

Fat-Loss-Food Cheat Sheet (*cont.*)

have high calorie density—in other words, a small portion has a lot of calories in it. It is, therefore, easy to overeat with a bowl of pasta. Not only that, but these foods can also disrupt blood sugar levels in susceptible people, leading to snacking and binging on less-desirable foods later.

Fatty desserts may fill us up in the moment, but they come with a very heavy calorie load, and new research is showing that these foods are not only difficult to stop eating once we start even if we are full, but also make us crave more of the exact same foods later. These foods are the worst ones to eat and should be eaten very rarely or sparingly.

Notice the two different lines on the chart? One depicts a typical reaction based on what we know from research on these foods' impact on satiety, as well as their calorie load. But the second line shows that this is certainly not a one-size-fits-all affair. Some may indeed get slightly better effects on HEC with lower-protein and higher-vegetable-and-starch diets. It is always important to filter food through your own metabolic expression (your individual responses to food, exercise, stress, and other factors). This is why being the detective is so critical. It's important to learn exactly what foods do and do not work for you.

The most satisfying macronutrient we have available to us is protein. In our attempt to control HEC, we turn to protein; otherwise the battle is lost from the beginning, and our metabolism never gets balanced. There's nothing wrong with wheat or dairy, but they are common allergens and if you have allergies to them, this can disrupt metabolic fat burning. We now know the immune system, hormone system, and nervous system are connected, so dysfunction in one can impact the others. This is why immune reactivity to foods can slow fat loss and cause metabolic dysfunction.

Tips on Starch

◎ Choose starches that are high in water, like oats, rice, quinoa, beans, and potatoes with the skin on.

◎ Avoid dry starches like breads, pastas, and chips.

Also, most people in the Western world are consuming a large proportion of their calories from wheat and dairy. Because of this, it's worth doing the detective work to see if eliminating these foods or dramatically reducing them helps your metabolic function. These foods could be hidden trigger foods that negatively impact your ability to lose weight. At the same time, don't believe the hype that they are a problem for all people. We're all different. You'll need to see for yourself. We also want to help you find your tolerance for starch and fat, so we take them out first, clearing the metabolic smoke, so to speak. If you choose to eliminate them completely, later, when you add them back in, you'll have the opportunity to clearly see how they affect you. The fat-loss game is a process and it takes time. We want you to find what works best for you. That's why we clean the slate to begin with, but now, if you feel you are ready, you can add some of these foods back in as you look to determine your individual tolerance.

To determine how fat and starch impact you as you search for the correct formula to keep your HEC in check, we ask you to watch fat and starch combinations on your plate. Remember that in the 4-2-2 approach, when you feed the lean, the ratio refers to the proportion of macronutrients on your plate. Four parts vegetable, two parts protein, two parts starch and/or fat. The reason we are making a point to say *starch and/or fat* is because typically that is where you will be doing your detective work. You will be trying to understand if fat or starch or both is most effective for you to keep HEC in check and get results. Some people may do better on starch and low fat. Some people are going to do better on high fat and low starch. Some people are going to have to find a happy medium between the two. That is the way we want you to begin thinking about food.

◎ Eat your starch last in each meal, after your veggies and protein are gone.

◎ Include vinegar-based dressings with your meals to help slow starch absorption.

◎ Spice your starches (see page 68), but avoid adding fat to them (unless that is the only thing that can keep your HEC in check).

Carbohydrates' Effects on HEC

Many people misunderstand carbs. All carbs are not the same, so let's stop talking about them like they are! There are nonstarchy and fiber-rich carbohydrates (vegetables), and there are high-water carbohydrates (like fruits and vegetables). There are high-starch and dry carbohydrates (like breads, crackers, chips, and cereals), and there are wet starches (like oatmeal, rice, potatoes, corn, and beans). Different varieties of carbs will have different effects on hunger, energy, and cravings. We want you to understand that for most people, the major foods that balance HEC are protein-, fiber-, and water-rich foods. These things satiate us. Among these foods are things like lean protein, vegetables, and lower-sugar fruits—fruits in general, really, because even the sugar in fruits is not a huge deal since there's so much water and fiber in fruits as well. Water helps fill us up faster and keep us full for longer and dilutes some of the sugar effect. The most challenging thing you will deal with is figuring out how the starchy stuff impacts you.

Tips on Vegetables

◎ Eat your veggies first in every meal to fill up before moving on to protein and then starches.

◎ Don't be afraid to add fat, salt, and spices to your vegetables.

◎ If you have sensitive digestion, make sure your veggies are well cooked.

◎ Whenever possible, start your meal with a salad and a vinegar-based dressing.

Tips on Fats

◎ Get your fats from fat-based foods and not as part of your protein.

◎ If you must eat fatty meats, buy or choose organic varieties to reduce persistent organic pollutants (POPs). They may still be there, but there will be fewer.

◎ Add fats to vegetables, not starches.

Fat-Loss Foods

Fat-loss foods are not something magical that you eat and they automatically make you lose fat. Rather, they are foods that help you control your HEC. We want you to eat fat-loss foods for this reason. Whenever you eat, you shut off fat burning, regardless of what it is that you eat. That's because food gives the body resources to burn *other* than its fat stores. So, when you focus on eating fat-loss foods, you'll likely eat less, since these foods make it very easy for you to go 4 to 6 hours after a meal without hunger, but with a balanced and predictable energy level, no cravings, great focus, a good mood, and high energy for your workouts. Fat-loss foods are rich in protein, fiber, and water—foods like lean protein and vegetables. Wet starches and fats can be fat-loss foods, too, but you have to figure out your individual tolerance for each. When some people eat too few starches, their HEC gets out of check. For example, they eat too much fat instead, and their HEC gets out of check, or they gain body fat. Some people will have eggs and bacon for breakfast and then crave fatty and sugary foods all day that day. So for them, that's not an effective nutrient combination to keep their HEC in check. But for others, the same breakfast gives lasting and sustained energy. If you think about it like that, this entire book is really trying to teach you that it's your job to figure out what's best for your body—and that one person's fat-loss food can be another's fat-storing food.

 ## COUNTING CALORIES

What we want you to *stop* thinking about so much is calories. The bottom line on calories is that you should *not* be obsessively counting them, although they do matter. Some of you, we know, have a psychological preference for numbers. Some of you don't. Either way, you do need to understand that calories matter.

Here's something to consider: We have patients who eat very-high-vegetable and very-high-protein diets. They live on salads and chicken and broccoli and

---

Dining Out on 4-2-2

Don't panic if you're eating out at a restaurant for dinner. Get a piece of grilled fish or chicken, ask for a side of steamed vegetables, and order a big salad with vinegar-based dressing. For your starch, choose a wet starch with high fiber— the added water makes these foods very satiating. Foods like rice, potatoes, quinoa, oats, and beans (our favorite) work best.

Eat More, Exercise More Protein Ratio Calculator

Just like in the ELEL stage, here's how to calculate your EMEM macronutrient intake for the numbers people out there (though we want you to get away from this sort of obsession!). This can, however, be a great guide from which to begin. The EMEM approach can create a calorie deficit or calorie surplus and be used for either weight loss or muscle gain. The amounts listed here are for weight loss primarily. Some may find they need to increase calorie and carb totals for muscle gain.

Always start by working out how many grams of protein you should eat and then calculating the calories and the amounts of the other macros from that.

◎ Set your protein grams to your weight in pounds. So a 200-pound person would be eating 200 grams of protein per day. If you weigh more than 200 pounds, 200 grams is the maximum protein intake, so set your level to 200 grams as well.

◎ Calculate the total calories using a 40:30:30 ratio of carbs to protein to fat. Remember, carbs increase insulin. And insulin is one of your best muscle-building hormones (i.e., it is anabolic). So insulin combined with weight training aids muscle gain.

So Jane, who weighs 200 pounds, will have a protein intake of 200 grams.

There are 4 calories per gram of protein.

4 × 200 = 800 calories of protein

From the number of calories of protein, you can calculate Jane's carbs and fat.

Now figure out how many calories 800 is 30 percent of. Dividing 800 by 0.30 gives Jane 2,666.66, or about 2,700 calories (we typically round up).

Now calculate Jane's carb calories.

2,700 × 0.40 = 1,080 calories of carbs

Remember that there are 4 calories per gram of carbs, so 1,080 ÷ 4 = 270 grams of carbs.

Now calculate Jane's fat calories. Remember, there are 9 calories per gram of fat.

**2,700 × 0.30 = 810, or 800
(we round down)**

800 ÷ 9 = 88.88, or 89 grams of fat

So the breakdown of Jane's calories and macronutrients per day is:

**2,700 calories
270 grams of carbs
200 grams of protein
89 grams of fat**

eggs and low-sugar fruits and little else. These people are often shocked to find that when they calculate their calories, they are in ranges that most people would define as extremely low. Yet they are happily and effortlessly maintaining those counts, and have high energy levels and effortless fat loss. That is ultimately what we want you to achieve for yourself. It is almost always the case that if you are eating high-protein, high-fiber, and water-based foods, your hormones will be balanced and your intake of calories will be low, resulting in effortless fat loss.

It is nearly impossible to overeat these high-protein, high-water, and fiber-rich foods, especially when they are low in fat and starch. Most of us overeat fat and starch. But on occasion, some people do find protein can have a negative impact on weight loss. If you are one of these types, and you have ruled out the fat that often comes along with animal foods as the culprit, then remember to always honor your individual metabolism and personal preferences. Just realize that if you are not going to be getting satiating protein, extra-high vegetable intake will likely be required.

Also, watch out for the *hidden sources* of calories that end up in protein shakes. Sometimes we find people are adding a lot of fruit, coconut oil, chia seeds, or some other high-calorie item to their protein shakes, making them 700-calorie drinks that cause weight gain. You can't go crazy adding fats and carbs to protein just because you think it's healthy for you. Just remember that for some, calorie

Meal Replacement versus Protein Shake

The protein shakes on this plan are simple: protein powder and unsweetened almond, coconut, or low-fat (1% or 2%) cow's milk or water. If you start adding carbs, fruits, sweeteners, fats, and other things to your shake, it becomes a meal replacement. When we advise you to drink a protein shake as a snack, be sure you're not creating a meal replacement, or you'll end up with a calorie excess. Skip the coconut oil, and skip the mango and other fruits. Stick to protein, ice if needed, and a low-calorie liquid. If you are going to add anything, we suggest you add a bit of pure fiber like apple pectin or psyllium. Adding this extra fiber duplicates the effects of a lean-protein-and-vegetable-based meal: protein, fiber, and water, with little starch or fat.

THE HEC CHECK

◎ Make sure your hunger is in check by always paying attention to protein, fiber, and water.

◎ Make sure your cravings are not an issue by watching that you are not going too low or too high in the amount of starch.

◎ Make sure your energy level is sustained and predictable by balancing the fats, carbs, and protein in each meal.

◎ Eating more frequently is beneficial for managing HEC when you are also exercising more.

counting may be required at times. It should always be used as a last resort, though, rather than a fundamental guide for the diet. That's why we warn people: Don't overdo it when adding extras to your shakes. Liquid meals are easy to overdo when they contain extra sugar and fat, even if those sugars and fats are considered "healthy" by the mainstream.

Ultimately, controlling fat and carb intake is going to yield the best results, and finding your individual tolerance is so important. While your protein intake will be less limited, remember that in your efforts to find hormonal balance, too much of anything can trigger a calorie surplus and thwart your efforts.

For sustained weight loss you need hormone balance (which we have covered in depth) and a calorie deficit. This is undisputed. You can achieve that in one of two ways: You can focus on calories first, or you can focus on quality first. We know from experience that the latter is most often successful for most people. We like the quality-first approach because usually it naturally and effortlessly leads to a calorie reduction, yet feels less depriving.

CAN I EAT TOO LITTLE?

Some clients ask us if they can eat too *little* on this plan. In a word: yes.

If you're losing fat but your HEC is *not* in check, you're in what we call the dieting state. If you've dieted in the past, you might be familiar with this state. A dieter is hungry and tired, yet she's forging on, fighting cravings left, right, and center. If you're ever there on this plan, increase your protein intake slightly. Drink water, eat fiber, and don't let yourself get hungry. (Hunger means you will likely binge later.) If that doesn't work, increase your starch intake slightly. Remember the goal here: HEC in check and hormones balanced. Fat can be burned, but without a HEC that's in check, your results will not be sustainable. Be a detective, not a dieter.

Think back to our earlier discussion of metabolic compensation. You want to steer clear of that, or you'll regain the weight you lost and likely add more. This state puts you on a metabolic credit card, and you'll pay later in pounds for sure. We don't want short-term results that hit you with a hefty penalty later. That's why most diets fail, why dieters get fatter, and why stubborn areas get more stubborn. Keeping HEC in check is critical.

THE 4-2-2 RECIPES

You can whip up just about anything at home that meets the requirements of the meals you'll be eating during this phase. During your two meals that contain starch, just remember the 4-2-2 ingredients and follow the plate—8 ounces of protein, ½ cup of starch, and veggies is a good starting place. Here are some of our breakfast favorites, but definitely try your own too. Some of these are from members of our team.

Breakfast Casserole by Emily Saunders

My husband and I made this for my family on Christmas morning last year to rave reviews. It's a perfect and simple way to feed a group of people on one dish in the morning. Enjoy!

½ pound breakfast sausage, turkey sausage, or leftover ground turkey

¼ cup chopped onion

1 large sweet potato, cubed

3 cups chopped spinach

1 cup chopped or finely chopped mushrooms

Leftover vegetables, such as broccoli, asparagus, etc.

3 cups egg whites or mixture of whole eggs and egg whites, whisked

2 ounces shredded regular or almond Cheddar cheese

Ground black pepper to taste

Paprika to taste

Preheat the oven to 350°F. Cook the sausage and onion in a skillet until no longer pink (if it's precooked, there's no need to reheat it). Microwave the sweet potato for 4 to 5 minutes. Coat a casserole dish with olive oil cooking spray and layer the meat evenly at the bottom. Add the sweet potatoes and veggies, and then the eggs. Sprinkle the cheese, pepper, and paprika on top. Bake for 35 to 50 minutes, or until browned to your liking.

SERVES 4

Per serving:
350 calories, 39g protein, 16g carbs, 4g fiber, 15g fat

Coconut Baked Oatmeal by Jillian Teta

Of late, I have been really excited about baked oatmeal. It may be nothing new to the health and fitness world, but it has opened up a whole new vista of yummy morning or postworkout meal options that feel super indulgent and are fast and easy. The core ingredients are egg whites, protein powder, and oats. From that base, the combinations and possibilities are endless and delightful. This recipe calls for a tantalizing combination of cocoa and coconut. I had this with a small glass of black iced coffee after running sprints. It was the first meal of the day.

6 egg whites

¾ cup filtered water

2 scoops protein powder

3 tablespoons unsweetened cocoa powder

½ cup old-fashioned rolled oats (or steel-cut oats)

2 tablespoons shredded coconut

3 teaspoons stevia, or to taste

2 dropperfuls liquid chocolate stevia (or another flavor, or more stevia)

3 drops coconut flavor (optional)

1 teaspoon apple cider vinegar

¼ teaspoon baking powder

Dash of vanilla

Pinch of sea salt

Preheat the oven to 350°F and coat a 9-by-9-inch glass baking dish with zero-calorie coconut oil cooking spray. Combine all ingredients in a blender and blend until smooth. Pour the mixture into the baking dish and sprinkle it with a bit of shredded coconut if desired. Bake until a knife inserted in the center comes out clean, 15 to 25 minutes, depending on your oven.

SERVES 2

Per serving:
300 calories, 41g protein, 26g carbs, 5g fiber, 4.5g fat

Gingerbread Protein Shake

8 ounces unsweetened vanilla-flavored almond milk

½ banana

¼ teaspoon ground cinnamon

⅛ teaspoon ground ginger

⅛ teaspoon ground nutmeg

Ice

Combine the milk, banana, cinnamon, ginger, and nutmeg in a blender. Add some ice and blend to desired consistency. Enjoy!

SERVES 1

Per serving:
230 calories, 27g protein, 24g carbs, 3g fiber, 3.5g fat

Blueberry–Chocolate Chip Pancakes

2 scoops protein powder

6 egg whites

½ cup steel-cut oats

1 tablespoon ground flaxseed

¼ teaspoon baking soda

¼ teaspoon baking powder

½ teaspoon apple cider vinegar

Pinch of sea salt

2 tablespoons chocolate chips

¼ cup fresh blueberries

Coconut nectar or sugar-free syrup to taste

Ground cinnamon

Heat a skillet over medium-high heat. Combine the protein powder, egg whites, oats, flaxseed, baking soda, baking powder, vinegar, and salt in a blender and blend to desired consistency. Fold in the chocolate chips and blueberries.

Coat the skillet with cooking spray and spoon ⅓ cup of batter per pancake into the skillet. Turn each pancake over when its edges are dry, after about 2 minutes, and cook the other side.

Top with coconut nectar or sugar-free syrup and a sprinkle of cinnamon. Enjoy!

SERVES 2

Per serving:
400 calories, 40g protein, 46g carbs, 7g fiber, 8g fat

OTHER BIOFEEDBACK CLUES

Because you'll be kicking your exercise up from the ELEL phase, we want you to pay close attention to your hunger and cravings and what outside factors impact them. Remember, cravings are impacted by stress hormones and almost always come from stress. Hunger is almost always related to either low food intake or low water intake. Hunger comes from the stomach; cravings are in the head. Boredom eating is usually a craving, and this kind of behavioral hunger is very different from biochemical hunger. If you can put bulk in your stomach to make you feel full, you can sometimes alleviate both.

Energy is a little trickier because it's impacted by many different things, but the area you have the most control over is blood sugar management. Insulin, cortisol, and adrenaline are the hormones that most impact blood sugar. Always pay attention to how stress and eating may help or hurt your blood sugar and energy levels.

Other biofeedback clues for assessing metabolic balance include:

◎ **Sleep and exercise recovery:** Paying attention to how your approach is impacting these activities will further help you know if your metabolism is out of control.

◎ **Mood:** Many things can impact your mood. Your brain chemicals play a strong role here. Dopamine is a brain chemical that makes you feel focused and alert. Serotonin makes you feel relaxed, confident, and appreciative. GABA makes you feel relaxed and able to easily recover after periods of stimulation or exertion. When the metabolism is balanced, your brain chemistry is more likely to be balanced (and vice versa). Changes in mood can be an early indicator of metabolic imbalance.

◎ **Digestion:** Digestion is a window into the balance between the sympathetic (fight or flight) and parasympathetic (rest and digest) nervous systems. Many doctors, including integrative doctors like us, refer to the digestive tract as the "second brain." This is because it has more neurons than anyplace except the brain. As you have learned, the immune, hormone, and nervous systems are interdependent and are constantly engaging in cross talk. This means that your digestive health gives you another unique window into metabolic function and health. Gas, bloating, heartburn, diarrhea, constipation, and irritable and inflammatory bowel issues are not separate from your fat-loss efforts—in fact, they are directly related to them. As you play detective and learn to assess your metabolic function, look to the GI tract as a key influencer on health, fitness, and fat loss.

◎ **Age:** Our metabolism is constantly changing. One of the main factors that changes metabolism is aging itself. That's why you need to stay on top of all of the factors listed here, so you can constantly adjust as needed. Some research does suggest that you can become insulin resistant as you age, and this may cause the slow rise in weight seen as we age. One of the benefits of learning to read the body's biofeedback is being able to know what the metabolism needs as you age. Once you learn the process of being a detective rather than a dieter, you will never be in the dark about what is required for metabolic balance.

Get Your HEC Back in Check in 3 Steps

Do some detective work to find the right adjustment.

Food

1. Raise protein, fiber, and water intakes.

2. Raise your fat intake slightly.

3. Raise your starch intake slightly.

Hunger versus Cravings

HUNGER	CRAVING
Increases over time	Is situational and habitual
Occurs in the gut (i.e., growling stomach)	Occurs in the head (e.g., taste for ice cream)
Occurs several hours after meals	Can happen anytime
Decreased by drinking water	Is not helped by water
Is satisfied by a meal	Is not satisfied by a meal
Can be suppressed by stress	Is activated by stress

Exercise

1. Walk more and do more low-intensity, long-duration exercise.

2. Decrease long-duration, moderate- to high-intensity exercise.

3. Find the right amount of short-duration, high-intensity exercise for you.

Lifestyle

1. Increase the amount of rest and recovery activities you are doing.

2. Use cocoa powder to stave off hunger and cravings.

3. Focus on controlling your behavioral and habitual eating by developing mindfulness about eating and your attitudes about food.

THE WORKOUT WINDOW

Eating your biggest, most starch-rich meal after you finish your workout is optimal. When you eat, insulin is released. Insulin increases the number of glucose receptors on all of your cells so they can get fed. Another way to do the same thing is with movement and exercise. Movement increases those same glucose receptors without insulin, so you are insulin sensitive in the first few hours after exercise. For that reason, the hours just after exercise are a great time to increase your intake of starchy foods to help tone muscle and feed the body. The process also helps in repair and recovery. An insulin-*sensitive* person who overeats calories—more specifically, carbs—is more likely to store them as muscle (and therefore not fat). An insulin-*resistant* person who overeats calories and carbs is more likely to store them as fat. This is the reason you should consume your starch-rich meals after a workout whenever possible.

Remember the myth of multitasking: The body can't build muscle and burn fat at the same time; instead, it likes to be either building muscle or burning fat. There are two exceptions to this rule. One is people just beginning to work out: They tend to be able to do both. The other is people using anabolic steroids (and we don't suggest that approach!). Just as you need a calorie deficit and hormonal balance to lose fat, you require calorie excess and hormonal balance to gain muscle. Muscle can't be gained in a time of calorie deficit. In order to gain muscle without storing fat, you need to be aware of how the metabolism functions. Honoring the Law of Metabolic Multitasking is important. Paying particular attention to the window of insulin sensitivity in the hours after intense exercise allows you to increase the chances you can both burn fat and build some muscle. This is the reason that in the 4-2-2 protocol, we call for more starch in the meals that come after your workout.

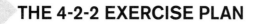

THE 4-2-2 EXERCISE PLAN

You'll be eating more in this phase, but exercising more as well.

Remember

- 4 metabolic chain workouts per week (20 minutes each)
- 2 rest-based interval training sessions per week (20 minutes each)
- 2 hours or more (about 20,000 steps) of leisurely walking on as many days as possible
- NOTE: If you are a runner, you may replace some of the walking with running. Just remember, this can easily be overdone and throw HEC out of check. So make sure it works for you. If it does, feel free to run instead of walk in two or three sessions during the week.

REST IS KEY

For both the metabolic chains and the interval training, you will be using a method of training we developed called rest-based training (RBT).

Rest and exercise are thought to be opposites, but they're actually complementary. In fact, the amount of resting you do during a workout determines how hard you can work. Think about it this way: A champion sprinter who attempts two 100-meter races one right after the other, without resting between them, could win the first race, but would likely finish last in the second race. The exertion required during the first race would be impossible to generate in the second.

Without rest, the sprinter could not physically or mentally compete. Resting between the races is required to reset the body. Only with rest could the sprinter

The Rest-Based Psychological Difference

Rest-based training uses rest, personal control, and time manipulation to optimize intensity for all fitness levels. Both the metabolic chain workouts and the rest-based interval training workouts use this technique. It combines the latest in exercise science and motivational psychology. Rest-based training has the same physiological benefits as intense interval exercise and weight training but also has unique psychological benefits.

The difference: Where interval training has clearly defined work and rest ratios, rest-based training leaves the exerciser in charge of when to rest and for how long. This shift acts as reverse psychology for exercisers, which is important considering how critical motivation is in terms of a person's ability to maintain consistency, frequency, and intensity. The primary goal of interval training is to maximize work effort across all work bouts and employ the shortest recovery time possible to maximize the training stimulus. Contrary to popular belief, research has shown that exercisers in control of their workouts often work harder and are able to self-regulate to the optimal work-to-rest ratio for their physiology. In this way, rest-based training is like interval training on steroids, yet at the same time it is safer and adaptable to all fitness levels.

push his or her body to its max a second time. The same applies to you and your workouts. By focusing attention on rest first, it is possible to achieve more high-quality work. Rest is not only a good thing—it's the primary goal of the training. The more you rest, the harder you will be able to push. The harder you push, the more rest you will require. Rest and work are synergistic: When used together intelligently, they deliver better results than can be achieved with standard "pace yourself" exercise.

When doing rest-based workouts, remember the phrase "Push until you can't, rest until you can." Some will prefer frequent short rest periods, while others may opt for longer periods of rest less often. With rest-based training, you use rest strategically to deliver just the right intensity for your individual metabolic needs. Push hard, rest hard, repeat: That is how these workouts deliver exceptional results.

Metabolic Conditioning

To understand the workouts in this section, you first have to understand that metabolic conditioning is *not* interval training. While you will be doing some interval exercise in this phase, metabolic conditioning is a bit different. Metabolic exercise is also very different from aerobic exercise. If the body is not being pushed to higher intensities than traditional aerobic exercise allows, you are not reaping the best benefits for your metabolism. These workouts are also not power lifting or bodybuilding. Both forms of exercise use long periods of rest, while metabolic conditioning has much shorter rest periods. If you take long rests between sets, are not feeling your chest pound, and are pacing yourself during long workouts, then you're not doing metabolic conditioning.

Finally, if you're engaging in what we call "circus workouts," which are workouts geared toward keeping you entertained instead of repeatedly attacking the same body parts again and again, you are missing the benefits of this style of training. Boot camps, for example, rarely produce the real benefits of metabolic conditioning.

When you are doing this style of training correctly, you will know it. It has a distinct feeling associated with it. If you have ever been in a tug-of-war battle, chopped wood, or pushed a heavy wheelbarrow up a hill, then you know how this training should feel—like hard but gratifying work. If not, we'll walk you through it and we're sure you'll feel it!

In these workouts you are doing both cardiovascular training and resistance training at the same time, and you will attack the same muscles again and again. Our patients describe this type of exercise as getting sucked into a vortex with a pair of dumbbells.

The Benefit

You'll balance your hormones, but also burn the maximum amount of calories possible during a workout. Metabolic conditioning also creates a metabolic ripple effect that produces elevated fat burning long after the workout has been completed. If the workout is done correctly to stimulate testosterone (more on that in a bit) and the diet has unlocked fat release, together they can ignite fat burning for days.

The Style

There are many different forms of high-intensity exercise, but our favorite, the one we used to design these workouts, was printed in the September 2008 issue of the *Journal of Strength and Conditioning Research*. This study compared two different versions of the same workout. In one version, the resistance training and cardiovascular portions were done separately, one after another. In the other version, the workout was done with the cardiovascular component inserted between sets of weight-lifting exercises. In other words, the second version merged the weight lifting and the cardiovascular exercise together. Despite using identical exercises and equal amounts of cardio and weight lifting in each version, the merged workout produced 10 times more fat loss than the other format.

The merged group also saw slightly better gains in muscle, and most fitness parameters also improved to a greater extent. The merged workout was able to deliver the benefits of both cardiovascular and weight-lifting exercises while also increasing the fat loss and improving muscle gains. Remember how we said building muscle and burning fat at the same time is very difficult for the body to do? Well, this style of workout makes it a bit easier.

The Mechanism

The results of the merged workout were impressive, but the special brand of metabolic-conditioning workouts we are going to introduce to you takes things one step further. The main difference: This workout uses relatively heavy weights, rather than having you do light machine exercises. The result: We'll deliver four stimulants to the metabolism, increasing the benefits of this type of workout. We call those stimulants the B's and the H's. The B's and H's will elevate your metabolic afterburn and release lactic acid, which might stimulate the release of growth hormone and testosterone, according to preliminary research.

- **Breathless.** You should be so breathless that you can't talk as you're exerting effort during the workout and are forced to rest at times because of it. You should be panting.

- **Burning.** You should reach metabolic failure, which is signaled by muscle burn so intense you need to stop and recover.

◎ **Heavy.** You need to lift weights heavy enough to induce strain in the muscles and joints at times. For this reason, you'll lift heavy weights and use explosive exercises like jumps and squats.

◎ **Heat.** This means you'll be getting hot and sweaty. Since we all sweat differently, this is the least effective biofeedback signal to assess during your workout. Increased heat means increased blood flow and therefore more fat being shuttled to the areas of the body that can burn it. You might find you sweat more as your fitness improves.

Exercise Recap

A few things to remember before we dive in to the specific workouts:

◎ Diet is still most important for fat loss, and exercise should never be overdone, especially in low-calorie states. Intense exercise can push the body into a state of muscle breakdown if done excessively over a period of time while dieting. Our workouts are designed in a way that forces the muscle to stay and the fat to burn away.

◎ Don't pace yourself in these workouts. Instead, use a rest-based "push until you can't, rest until you can" format: Push hard, then rest until you can push hard again. The workout is short for a reason: The longer a workout is, the more likely you will be to pace yourself. Twenty minutes of doing this type of workout at full intensity will outperform hourlong workouts done the "old-fashioned" way. We have seen this over and over again in clinical practice.

◎ Our version of metabolic conditioning is individualized. Everyone's sweet spot is a little different. This is why one-size-fits-all circuits with defined rest periods are not as effective as rest-based training. In order to get the proper response, rest just long enough to be able to push hard a second time.

Metabolic Physique Conditioning

Our specific brand of metabolic conditioning involves overloading the muscles. We call it Metabolic Physique Conditioning. Metabolic conditioning is wonderful at burning fat, but it can fall short in muscle toning unless it's tweaked somewhat. In order to make sure you are getting the best of both worlds, our metabolic chain workouts add in more of a muscle-building approach. This adds what exercise coaches call overload. *Overload* means that for the body to respond it must again and again encounter an increasingly greater stimulus that forces it to adapt. This is why you must do more than one set of exercises, increase your weights frequently, and make sure the muscles you are working are actually stimulated again and again. When we look at the way fitness training is currently done, we are appalled by the lack of overload being employed. If you want exercise to enhance the look of your physique and help burn stubborn fat, then you must embrace this concept.

How Does It Work?

Here are the aspects of the Metabolic Physique Conditioning workouts you will be doing. We want you to understand why we built them the way we did.

◎ **Short rests.** Keeping rest periods short means the workout intensity can be elevated to adequately generate the B's and H's.

◎ **Full-body exercises.** Using full-body exercises that involve multiple planes of movement not only adds to the metabolic elements of the workout, but also develops greater fitness and a more athletic-looking physique. We are not going for big and bulky or skinny fat; we are going for the athletic look. Full-body exercises are also the best way to merge the cardio component into a weight-training workout.

◎ **Overload.** To get individual muscles to respond, they must encounter overload. Multiple sets and reps of the same movements will always be used in these workouts to achieve this effect.

◎ **Rest-based training.** This approach is an essential tool in these workouts. The workouts literally can't be done without it. Using structured rest periods ignores the individual metabolism and fitness level, causing many to miss out on the workout's benefits. The idea is to optimize your work-to-rest ratio.

THE METABOLIC CHAIN WORKOUTS

For each chain:

◎ Choose a weight that allows a 10-rep max on the weakest movement in a workout (whichever movement is most difficult for you and requires the lowest weight). For example, in the burpee chain, the weakest movement is the curl.

In the incline chain, the weakest movement is the side raise. In the leg chain, the weakest movement is the squat jump. Choose your dumbbells based on those moves.

◎ Set your watch, and time the exercise—you will be going for 20 minutes straight.

◎ Use the RBT method and rest whenever you need to, especially if you are losing form or approaching metabolic or mechanical failure. Rest for as long as you require and then start the workout again as soon as you are able to. Start right where you left off. The clock keeps ticking whether you are working or resting.

◎ To begin, do 1 rep of each exercise in the chain. On your second round, do 2 reps of each exercise; on the third round, do 3 reps of each; and so on.

◎ After your fifth round, start back at 1 rep per exercise and work your way back up the chain to 5 again.

◎ Try to complete as many chains as possible in the allotted time, and take note of how many you complete to track your progress.

See page 124 for a sample workout diagram explaining this unique workout.

The Metabolic Chain

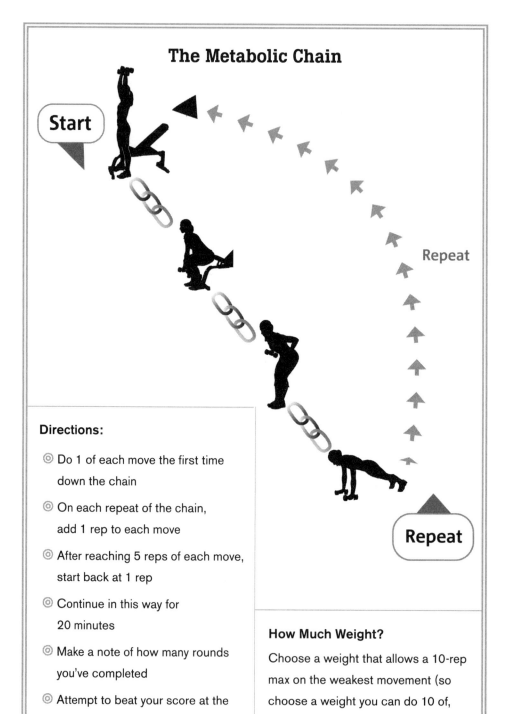

Start

Repeat

Repeat

Directions:

- ◎ Do 1 of each move the first time down the chain
- ◎ On each repeat of the chain, add 1 rep to each move
- ◎ After reaching 5 reps of each move, start back at 1 rep
- ◎ Continue in this way for 20 minutes
- ◎ Make a note of how many rounds you've completed
- ◎ Attempt to beat your score at the next workout

How Much Weight?

Choose a weight that allows a 10-rep max on the weakest movement (so choose a weight you can do 10 of, but not 11).

WORKOUT 1: THE BURPEE CHAIN

WEIGHTED BURPEE / PUSHUP / BENT-OVER ROW / CURL / PRESS

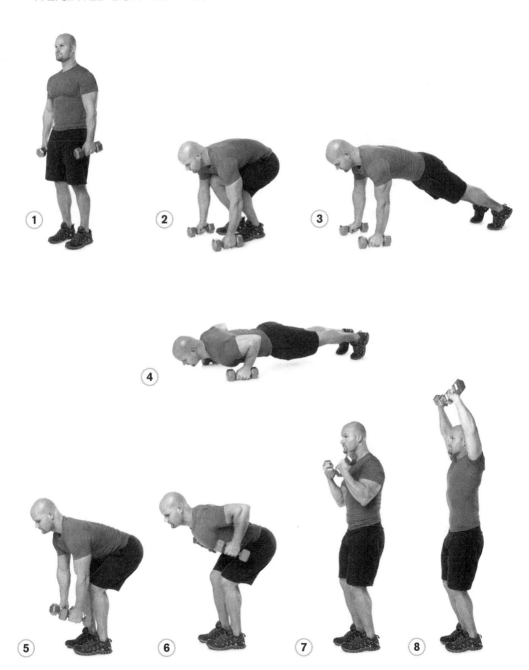

WORKOUT 2: THE LEG CHAIN

LUNGE (RIGHT LEG) / SQUAT / LUNGE (LEFT LEG) / SQUAT JUMP

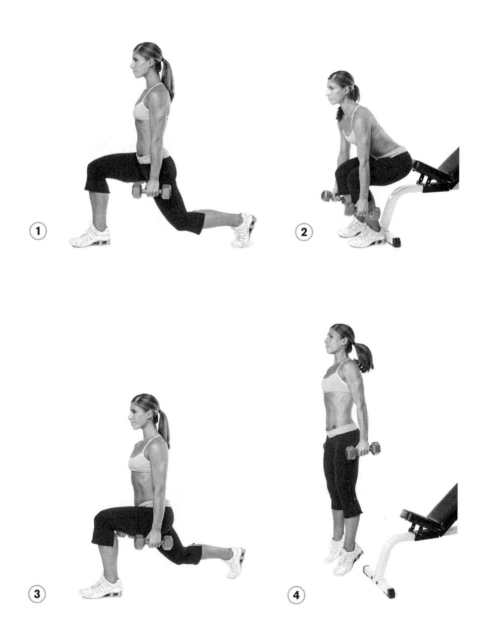

WORKOUT 3: THE INCLINE CHAIN

INCLINE CURL / PRESS / LUNGE (RIGHT LEG) / ROW /
LUNGE (LEFT LEG) / SIDE RAISE

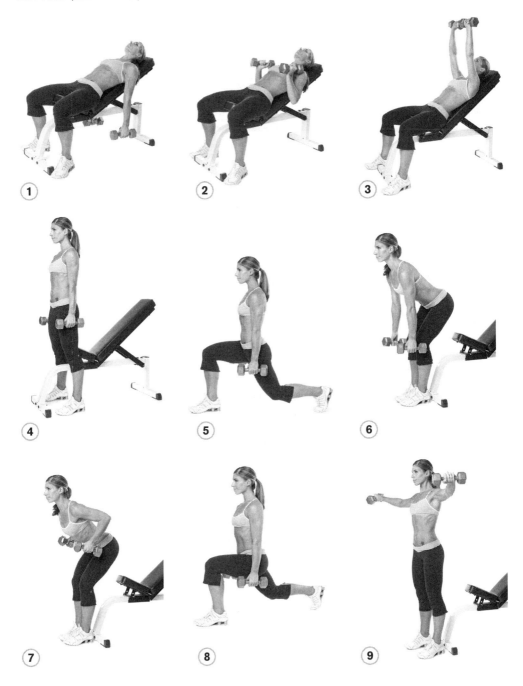

REST-BASED INTERVAL TRAINING (RBIT)

Twice per week. Compared to traditional interval workouts, we believe our intervals are more effective, safer, and individualized. We want you to push as hard as possible, then rest as long as needed. The work intervals are set; the rest intervals are not. We're putting the control in your hands instead of telling you how much rest you need between bouts to be ready to go again. Don't try to be tough, either: We really want you to rest, literally to move in slow motion until you feel 100 percent ready to exert yourself at high intensity again.

As you do in the metabolic chain workouts, you will focus on time, not the number of intervals you complete. You'll do as many interval rounds as you can complete in a 20-minute span. You'll be able to notice improvement, and you won't dread the workout because you're in charge.

Rest-based intervals are our form of individualized interval training that adapts to all fitness levels. Feel free to use any piece of cardio equipment or even a track, steps, or a patch of flat road or grass. These can even be done at home in a small area by doing high knees or jumping jacks, jumping rope, or using a mountain climber or any other cardio-based or callisthenic exercise aimed at the cardiovascular system.

Here is the protocol to be done twice a week in the 4-2-2 phase.

◎ 5-minute warmup doing a low-intensity version of the exercise for the workout:

- 20-second full-exertion sprint followed by slow-motion rest as long as is required

- 30-second full-exertion sprint followed by slow-motion rest as long as is required

- 40-second full-exertion sprint followed by slow-motion rest as long as is required

- 60-second full-exertion sprint followed by slow-motion rest as long as is required

- Repeat this sequence for 20 minutes, completing as many rounds as possible.

◎ 5-minute cooldown

CYCLE THE DIET

To achieve the results you are looking for, start cycling the diet, doing the ELEL phase for 2 weeks and then switching to the EMEM phase for 2 weeks. Continue cycling until you reach your desired weight. Remember: The only way to do this is to become a fat-loss detective—you will need to practice and master the tenets of the plan over time. Just like if you were learning a new language or how to play an instrument, you do not get to cheat your way to a brand-new body. This is a journey. For some, this could go on for months, while for others a few cycles is all that is required for the desired results. You'll then move into the maintenance part of this plan, which will ensure your long-term success.

THE LOSE WEIGHT HERE RECAP

◎ While it's nearly impossible to overeat protein- and fiber-based foods, calories still matter.

◎ Find your unique tolerance for fats and starches. There is nothing wrong with either, but they can lead to problems, especially when combined.

◎ Food is information for the body. One person's fat-loss food is another person's fat-gaining food. Your job is to understand how food impacts HEC and your other biofeedback signals as well as how it impacts fat storage.

◎ Find your nutritional approach using the structured plan we have provided to get you started, but remember to be flexible and adjust according to your individual metabolic reactions, psychology, and personal preferences.

◎ After completing the EMEM phase for 2 weeks, start the ELEL phase again and alternate the two until you reach your desired results. At that point, move on to the maintenance phase, outlined in the next chapter.

Kelly

Kelly looked good on the outside, but inside she was a self-proclaimed mess. A fitness instructor for 18 years, Kelly was always exhausted. Maintaining her fit and lean physique left her overtrained, sleep-deprived, eating too little, and exercising too much. The result was emotional strain and major stress.

When Lose Weight Here came along, everything changed for Kelly. She became a diet detective and worked to finally figure out her own metabolism and what was best for her. She started

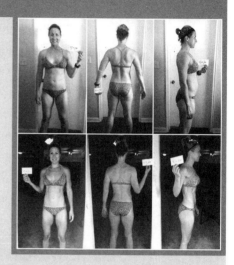

to feel really good, despite an initial panic she wouldn't be working out enough. Eventually, the stress of her life eased. She began sleeping better and found an overall sense of calm. Also, after cycling her diet through the varying phases and doing heavy weights and walking, she went from being "puffy-fit" down 12 pounds and several inches, looking great.

CHAPTER 7

MAINTENANCE:

Transform Your Body for Good

First of all, congratulations for reaching this point! You've accomplished your goals, you're at a weight and size you love, you feel strong and fit, and you've figured out how to keep your hunger-energy-cravings (HEC) in check. The work isn't over, because this is the body you want to live in for life. You've done the diet detective work and figured out what works, but now it's time to keep your metabolism working for you so you can maintain this wonderful new you. You'll do this by building on what you have already learned and practicing until it becomes second nature.

The maintenance phase adheres to the principles laid out in the Eat Less, Exercise Less (ELEL) and Eat More, Exercise More (EMEM) phases but gives you more eating and exercising choices, which makes it easier to stick to for life. Essentially, during the week you'll do a modified ELEL fat-blasting plan, coupled with a modified muscle-toning EMEM program on the weekends. You will eat more on the weekends when you are more active, which is what most people's schedules allow for.

HOW DO YOU KNOW WHEN IT'S TIME TO MAINTAIN?

Let's make sure you're where you want to be. Typically, our patients need 2 to 4 weeks minimum in the 3-2-1 repair phase to starve the fat, repair some of the metabolic damage from dieting, and get the metabolism ticking again. In the 3-2-1 and 4-2-2 cycling phase, we have observed that a 2- to 3-month period is needed. For some, results aren't fully realized until the 6-month mark. Again, we're all wired differently and it will take a different formula and amount of time for each of us to get to this stage. As a rule of thumb, we suggest cycling between 3-2-1 and 4-2-2 for a total of 12 weeks. And it doesn't end there. Many people still achieve often unexpected fat loss in the maintenance phase.

TIME TO MAINTAIN

Let's review a little about where you have been. Remember how this all began? You realized that your metabolism does not function the way you thought it did. By treating your metabolism like a calculator for all those years, you got caught in the diet trap. We reversed the damage of dieting and you learned to build a plan that worked with rather than against your metabolism.

You also made a critical shift in mind-set from that of a dieter to that of a detective using the AIM process to Assess, Investigate, and Modify. That process doesn't end here. In fact, it ramps up to some degree so all of your hard work lives on. You will continue monitoring HEC and assessing changes in your body composition and shape, as well as practicing the investigation and modification processes. This is a lifelong endeavor, and practicing it will soon be second nature.

Regularly Check In with Yourself

◎ Is your HEC still in check?

◎ Are you continuing to burn fat?

Also, be careful not to overdo it. Don't get so excited about the results that you ramp them up by working out more or eating less. Stay the course, follow the plan, don't try to overachieve. If things are working, stick with it.

Measure Each Week

First thing every Friday morning, take your measurements, weigh yourself, and check your status—forever more. Keep on top of it, especially in the initial stages of maintenance. This will serve as a valuable check-in so you don't gain back any or all of the weight you lost by throwing your hands in the air and reverting to your old habits. Continue to assess yourself on Fridays so you'll have a basic understanding of what increasing your eating on weekends does for your weight.

MAINTENANCE STRATEGY: WEEKEND-WARRIOR MODE

Ideally, most of you will get into the weekend-warrior mode for life: Eat Less, Exercise Less during the week and Eat More, Exercise More on the weekend. It's as simple as that. It's an efficient structure to follow and it fits in with most people's Monday-to-Friday work regimen. We take that approach because that's sort of how we all live our lives anyway: We work hard at our jobs and our lives during the week, and we kick back on the weekends and try to enjoy things a bit more, leaving the day-to-day stresses at the office.

Monday Morning through Friday Afternoon

◎ Keep it simple: Continue to use the shakes if they work for you, and keep up the walking to keep your hormones aligned.

◎ Eat your regular healthy meal following the 3-2-1 proportions at dinnertime.

◎ Continue to prioritize rest and relaxation.

Friday Night, Saturday, and Sunday

◎ You'll likely be eating out and doing more social activities. Enjoy this time and relax.

◎ Ramp up your exercise to make this a lifestyle that keeps your results stable or even improves upon them.

◎ You don't need to go crazy with exercise. Just realize that you will want to do something that pushes any extra calories you take in on the weekend into fueling your exercise or maintaining and toning lean muscle. This means weight training is your best bet. Use the metabolic chain workouts and/or the traditional weight-training workouts we have already taught you.

◎ On Friday night and on Saturday and Sunday, we want you to eat what you want. That's where the free meal comes into play. What does that mean specifically? Well, it means different things to all of us. But the easiest way to think about this is to just eat 100 percent freely, without limitations, at one to three meals during the weekend. This could be a Friday night out for drinks with friends, a Saturday afternoon burger or pizza while watching the games, or a Sunday pancake brunch with the girls. You may find doing this one time is more than adequate and any more than that causes you to slip back, or you may find you can easily do three meals in this fashion and notice great results. Limit this meal to a 2-hour time frame to keep yourself from eating continually all day.

Let's say you start maintenance thinking you can have a cheat meal on Friday night and Saturday night. You order pizza, you eat Chinese food, and you have more wine than usual. If that works for you, and 1 month into this phase you are still looking great and feeling great, then by all means, we encourage you to enjoy. If, however, those pants you worked so hard to fit into start getting tight again, then you've overdone it and will need to scale back. Maybe try to adjust those cheat meals somewhat, making one thing on your plate a cheat and filling the rest with salad and veggies. Maybe wine or dessert ends up being your only cheat. Maybe you are only able to handle one cheat night instead of two. Maybe adjust what a cheat night means to you. Maybe it just means wine with dinner. Maybe it means one slice of pizza and a big salad. Maybe it means a regular 3-2-1 meal, plus dessert. Being a diet detective is a lifelong practice even at this stage, so you'll need to figure out what works and adjust accordingly. Do what works, and always observe and adjust.

What's a Cheat Meal?

A cheat meal can be anything: fondue, pizza, burgers, or even beer. It's anything you want within a 2-hour time frame. To get extra muscle-toning benefits from these meals, try to eat them within a few hours after intense exercise, like weight training.

DO WHAT WORKS FOR YOU

We'd like to think 3-2-1 during the week and 4-2-2 on weekends works for us all, but the fact remains, it simply may not work for you. You may need to adjust the structure of your maintenance plans to accommodate your metabolism, psychology, and preferences. There are several approaches to consider when you use the weekend-warrior mode as the starting point and work backward from there as needed.

Diet Detective: Varied Approaches

1. **The Weekend Warrior:** Eat Less, Exercise Less on Monday through Friday. On the weekend, follow the same approach, but instead of one regular meal at the end of each day, eat a large cheat meal one to three times during the weekend. At the same time, make sure you get in a few weight-training workouts and maybe a long run or bike ride. This strategy puts you in the Eat Less, Exercise Less approach during the week and the Eat More, Exercise More framework on the weekend. Trial and error, as well as flexibility, are key to seeing if this will work for you.

2. **The Weekend Couch Potato:** Eat More, Exercise More Monday through Friday, and then on the weekend eat sparingly while engaging in light or no activity.

3. **The Exerciser:** Set your exercise schedule for the week and eat more on the days you exercise. Eat less on recovery days. For those who love exercise, this approach works best and is the lifestyle many will naturally gravitate to. It works well because you learn to instinctively match intake with output.

4. **The Lazy Girl or Boy:** Can you live on 3-2-1? Many can. In fact, this is the way many Europeans live, and probably the way your great-grandparents did, too. They were not running around like crazy, exercising like they were going mad. They ate sparingly and they moved a lot, but they did not exercise much. So, yes, that's something to consider at this phase. If it works for you and your HEC stays in check, then you can make

this your ongoing approach aside from the occasional period of eating more and moving less or eating less and moving more.

5. **The Athlete:** Maybe the 4-2-2 approach is your sweet spot. You are active every single day and need to fuel your body to keep it going. The people who live this lifestyle tend to have the bodies we admire the most. They train hard, they fuel smart, and they have lean, functional, athletic physiques. The only drawback to this lifestyle is what happens if the movement stops due to injury or just life catching up. Because some of these types have never really learned how their metabolism works, many end up gaining weight quickly because they are thrust into an Eat More, Exercise Less state. Then when they seek advice from the average everyday health professional, they will be told eat less and exercise more to lose the weight. If they follow this advice, they often inadvertently get caught in the diet trap with the rest of us, forgetting the rule of matching intake and output the way they functioned as athletes. Since you have been educated by this book, that is not a mistake you will make. You now know better. With all of this in mind, you can stay in this state, perhaps with brief breaks from it when on vacation.

The diet detective in you will help you figure out which of these works best for you. It may take some trial and error, but you'll get there. Be flexible. Life will have you moving through many of these stages at some point, or one may just work better for you all the time. Here are some weekly sample plans.

The Weekend Warrior

DAY	MEAL 1	MEAL 2	MEAL 3	EXERCISE	R&R
Monday	Protein smoothie or high-protein and vegetable meal	Protein smoothie or high-protein and vegetable meal	Salmon, kale, brown rice	1–2 hour leisurely walk (about 5,000–10,000 steps)	Hot Epsom salts bath
Tuesday	Protein smoothie or high-protein and vegetable meal	Large convenience salad with chicken, mixed greens, and vinegar dressing	Bison and bean chili	1–2 hour leisurely walk (about 5,000–10,000 steps)	
Wednesday	Veggie frittata	Protein smoothie or high-protein and vegetable meal	Grilled chicken breast, sweet potato, vegetable medley	1–2 hour leisurely walk (about 5,000–10,000 steps)	Sauna time
Thursday	Protein smoothie or high-protein and vegetable meal	Protein smoothie or high-protein and vegetable meal	Chicken veggie stir-fry, white rice	1–2 hour leisurely walk (about 5,000–10,000 steps)	
Friday	Protein smoothie or high-protein and vegetable meal	Protein smoothie or high-protein and vegetable meal	4 slices pepperoni pizza, 3 beers	Weight training	
Saturday	Protein smoothie or high-protein and vegetable meal	Protein smoothie or high-protein and vegetable meal	Mexican restaurant: chips and salsa, chicken fajita, margarita	2-hour bike ride	
Sunday	Restaurant brunch: eggs, bacon, hash browns	Protein smoothie or high-protein and vegetable meal	Large mixed green salad with chicken	Weight training	

Notice how the Weekend Warriors follow a very structured, convenience-oriented 3-2-1 approach during the week. During the weekend, they do not vary this approach much in terms of meal frequency, but they do significantly alter their food intake, and you will see them eating several very heavy meals that combine lots of fat, sugar, and salt and alcohol. At the same time, though, they exercise more on the weekend, so many of those extra calories will go into fueling exercise and building muscle. Obviously, if they are using this approach as a lifestyle, they have learned to circumvent some of the negative brain chemistry effects the weekend junk foods might have.

The Weekend Couch Potato

DAY	MEAL 1	MEAL 2	MEAL 3	MEAL 4	EXERCISE	R&R
Monday	Scrambled eggs, blueberries	Large salad with chicken	Postworkout recovery shake with added banana	Skirt steak, broccoli, cauliflower, boiled potatoes	30 minutes of high-intensity mixed cardio and weight training, 30 minutes of self-massage (using a foam roller) and mobility work	
Tuesday	Protein smoothie or high-protein and vegetable meal	Large convenience salad with chicken, mixed greens, and vinegar dressing	Postworkout recovery shake with added banana	Black bean chicken soup	30 minutes of high-intensity mixed cardio and weight training, 30 minutes of self-massage (using a foam roller) and mobility work	
Wednesday	Veggie frittata	Grilled chicken breast, vegetable medley	Postworkout recovery shake with added banana	Leftover grilled chicken, broccoli, brown rice	30-minute sprint intervals	
Thursday	Leftover grilled chicken, broccoli, brown rice	Chicken veggie stir-fry, white rice	Protein smoothie or high-protein and vegetable meal	Salmon, spinach salad, mixed squash medley	3-mile run	
Friday	Scrambled eggs, Canadian bacon	Large salad with chicken	Restaurant sushi, wine		None	Funny movie
Saturday	Black coffee	Protein smoothie or high-protein and vegetable meal	Takeout pizza		None	Hot Epsom salts bath
Sunday	Black coffee	Protein smoothie or high-protein and vegetable meal	Large mixed green salad with chicken		None	Long nap

Notice how in this scenario the week is loaded with exercise and therefore there are more meals, and that those meals include healthier starchy carbs in the meals after workouts to help with exercise recovery and muscle development. This is very similar to a 4-2-2 approach. But then the weekend is very light on food. The person is eating what they like but taking it easy, and opts to sleep in and fast until lunch. Doing things this way allows you to have a very relaxing weekend with less food and activity.

The Exerciser

DAY	MEAL 1	MEAL 2	MEAL 3	MEAL 4	EXERCISE	R&R
Monday	Scrambled eggs, blueberries, oats	Protein smoothie with added banana	Large salad with chicken	Skirt steak, broccoli, cauliflower	30 minutes of high-intensity mixed cardio and weight training, 30 minutes of self-massage (using a foam roller) and mobility work	
Tuesday	Protein smoothie or high-protein and vegetable meal	Large convenience salad with chicken, mixed greens, and vinegar dressing	Black bean chicken soup			Hot Epsom salts bath
Wednesday	Veggie frittata	Grilled chicken breast, sweet potato, vegetable medley	Postworkout recovery shake with added banana	Salmon fillet, broccoli, brown rice	30-minute sprint intervals	
Thursday	Leftover salmon fillet, broccoli, brown rice	Protein smoothie or high-protein and vegetable meal	Pork chop, spinach salad, mixed squash medley			1–2 hour leisurely walk (about 5,000–10,000 steps)
Friday	Scrambled eggs, Canadian bacon, cream of rice, mixed fruit	Protein smoothie with added banana	Large salad with chicken, vegetable soup	Filet, broccoli, wine	1-hour metabolic conditioning workout	Funny movie
Saturday	Scrambled eggs, oatmeal, Greek yogurt, mixed fruit	Postworkout recovery shake with added banana	Large burrito bowl with extra veggies (no rice or beans)	Spaghetti squash and meatballs, red wine	1 hour of weight training	
Sunday	Black coffee	Protein smoothie or high-protein and vegetable meal	Large mixed green salad with chicken		None	Massage

In this scenario, on the days when exercise is done, the meal frequency, carbohydrates, and calorie counts are increased. On the days when there is no exercise, the food intake is lower and there are fewer meals. This is a very intuitive approach, and one many will gravitate to as they master the rule of matching food intake with output.

The Lazy Girl or Boy

DAY	MEAL 1	MEAL 2	MEAL 3	EXERCISE	R&R
Monday	Protein smoothie or high-protein and vegetable meal	Protein smoothie or high-protein and vegetable meal	Salmon, kale, brown rice	Weight training	Hot Epsom salts bath
Tuesday	Protein smoothie or high-protein and vegetable meal	Large convenience salad with chicken, mixed greens, and vinegar dressing	Bison, bean chili	1–2 hour leisurely walk (about 5,000–10,000 steps)	
Wednesday	Veggie frittata	Protein smoothie or high-protein and vegetable meal	Grilled chicken breast, sweet potato, vegetable medley	Weight training	Sauna time
Thursday	Protein smoothie or high-protein and vegetable meal	Protein smoothie or high-protein and vegetable meal	Chicken veggie stir-fry, white rice	1–2 hour leisurely walk (about 5,000–10,000 steps)	
Friday	Protein smoothie or high-protein and vegetable meal	Protein smoothie or high-protein and vegetable meal	Large salad, 2 glasses of wine	1–2 hour leisurely walk (about 5,000–10,000 steps)	
Saturday	Protein smoothie or high-protein and vegetable meal	Protein smoothie or high-protein and vegetable meal	Large green chopped salad with salmon	1–2 hour leisurely walk (about 5,000–10,000 steps)	
Sunday	Black coffee	Protein smoothie or high-protein and vegetable meal	Large mixed green salad with chicken	1–2 hour leisurely walk (about 5,000–10,000 steps)	

In this scenario, 3-2-1 is followed indefinitely. You will notice the wine on Friday night and the skipping of the first meal on Sunday. That's because these people are not expending that much energy and therefore do not require lots of calories. You will also notice how protein is used and weight training is still done only two times a week. They understand that as they age, holding on to their muscle mass is imperative for the health of their metabolism, so they are making that a priority.

The Athlete

DAY	MEAL 1	MEAL 2	MEAL 3	MEAL 4	EXERCISE	R&R
Monday	Protein smoothie or high-protein and vegetable meal	Large salad with chicken	1 can of tuna, celery, baked potato	Skirt steak, broccoli, cauliflower, boiled potatoes	30 minutes of high-intensity mixed cardio and weight training, 30 minutes of self-massage (using a foam roller) and mobility work	
Tuesday	Protein smoothie or high-protein and vegetable meal	Large convenience salad with chicken, mixed greens, and vinegar dressing	Postworkout protein shake with added banana	Stir-fry with mixed vegetables, chicken, rice	1–2 hour leisurely walk (about 5,000–10,000 steps)	Hot Epsom salts bath
Wednesday	Veggie frittata	Grilled chicken breast, vegetable medley	Postworkout protein shake with added banana	Beef tips, broccoli, brown rice	30-minute sprint intervals	
Thursday	Leftover beef tips, broccoli, brown rice	Protein smoothie or high-protein and vegetable meal	Chicken, mashed sweet potato, vegetables	Salmon, spinach salad, mixed squash medley, quinoa	30 minutes of high-intensity mixed cardio and weight training, 30 minutes of self-massage (using a foam roller) and mobility work	1-hour leisurely walk (about 10,000 steps)
Friday	Scrambled eggs, Canadian bacon, cream of rice	Postworkout protein shake with added banana	Large salad with chicken	Beef filet, brussels sprouts, wine	1-hour metabolic conditioning workout	Funny movie
Saturday	Scrambled eggs, turkey sausage, mixed berries	Large mixed green salad, shrimp cocktail	Postworkout protein shake with added banana	Pasta and meatballs, red wine	1 hour of weight training	
Sunday	(brunch): Eggs, pancakes, hash browns, bacon	Protein smoothie or high-protein and vegetable meal	Large mixed green salad with chicken		None	Massage

In this scenario, intense activity is done every day except Sunday, and as a result these people are eating frequently, making judicious use of supplemental protein, and not cutting calories. Notice that on Sunday there is a very large brunch meal. Given the large amount of activity, this very-high-calorie meal will likely go toward recovery and have little negative effect on fat gain. This reflects what a typical athlete's eating and exercise regimens might look like.

THE FOUR METABOLIC TOGGLE SWITCHES

Our patients share a lot of stories with us about "slipping up" or "over-enjoying" a vacation. I (Jade here) went to London recently, and while I set out to follow Eat Less, Exercise Less because I had jam-packed days of lecturing scheduled, I ended up indulging in the great Indian food, fish and chips, and English beer London has to offer. I ate more and I exercised less. I ended up gaining a few pounds on my trip. Still, this Eat More, Exercise Less approach can in some instances be beneficial for your metabolism. Remember, the metabolism is built to compensate and adjust. Any change you make to eating and exercise can help you adjust back to the right direction if you know how to do it. And life makes it so you will eventually encounter times that are naturally unpredictable anyway. You can't always follow ELEL or EMEM.

That's one of the things we want to introduce you to at this point: the four metabolic toggle switches. You have worked really hard to understand that the Eat Less, Exercise More approach, when repeated over and over again or taken to the extreme, is not healthy for the metabolism. You also intuitively know that the standard Western couch potato lifestyle (or trips to London!) of eating more and exercising less can quickly cause weight gain and damage your health. And at this stage, while Eat Less, Exercise Less and Eat More, Exercise More have worked well for you, it is useful to know that the other two strategies can also be useful instruments in your metabolic toolbox.

Cycling the diet in any of the four directions can help to circumvent metabolic compensation. You can think of these four approaches as metabolic toggle switches. When the body compensates and weight loss stalls, you switch one toggle off and another one on. We've given you two: ELEL and EMEM. Since your work, family, and leisure activities keep your schedule changing, we know the other two toggles—Eat Less, Exercise More and Eat More, Exercise Less—will also be a part of your life, and this can actually be beneficial if you know how to use them intelligently. Now that your metabolism is healed and you know how to read the way your metabolism works, you'll likely find life will present different challenges. Knowing there is benefit to switching toggles at times means you don't have to stress as much. So long as your metabolism is healthy and these changes are short lived, they can be extremely beneficial and are one of the best ways to break through a plateau. You're an experienced diet detective at this point, and you'll know how to handle the shift from toggle to toggle and when it is time to move from one to another.

Here's a chart showing the four toggles along with the goal or outcome that results from each one. Both EMEM and ELEL are great for fat loss, but EMEM is a little better if you want to focus on muscle gain as well.

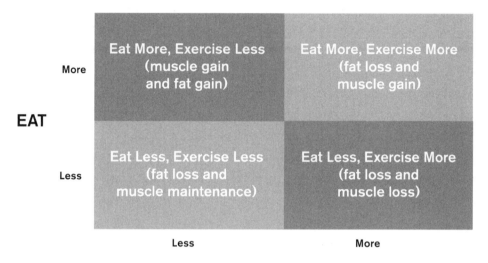

EAT

More — Eat More, Exercise Less (muscle gain and fat gain) — Eat More, Exercise More (fat loss and muscle gain)

Less — Eat Less, Exercise Less (fat loss and muscle maintenance) — Eat Less, Exercise More (fat loss and muscle loss)

Less   More

EXERCISE

All these options work because the metabolism is adaptive and reactive. Typically when you expose it to something new, it will respond for a time before adapting and then pushing back against you. So long as you have learned to read the signs, you can use this to your advantage. Eat Less, Exercise Less and Eat More, Exercise More are far safer and much more stable tools for long-term body change. This is because they can create the calorie deficit you need and are better at keeping the metabolism balanced. With the other two strategies, you need to be far more careful, but using them to your advantage for short periods of time and as a convenient means of adjusting to lifestyle situations can be useful. The point is to learn to use these strategies while being fully aware that you are doing so, without it taking much mental effort on your part. Done right, it should all begin to happen intuitively, and you will soon be one of those types who instinctively adjusts their approach on the fly and remains thin and lean as a result. As we have done throughout, we will provide some structure, and then you can adapt your approach to fit your needs.

The Busy Executive: Rotate Phases on Your Schedule

Here's an example: Let's say you are a busy executive and you travel frequently. You have periods of time when you are home for a stretch and then other times when you are on the road. Maybe it is easier for you to follow a very simple 3-2-1 Eat Less, Exercise Less plan while you travel. But when you are home and can do a different routine, you have access to your gym and like to exercise. At this stage you may choose to follow an Eat More, Exercise More approach. Now let's say you take a vacation for a long weekend and you want to go hiking, biking, running, sailing, rock climbing—you name it—but you don't really want to bother yourself too much about food. You decide to use this as a great time to switch to the Eat Less, Exercise More toggle. After all, it is only for a few days and you have learned to decipher whether you are getting into metabolic compensation. Finally, the holidays roll around and you are at home with the family. Lots of meals, a ton of socializing, no access to your gym, and it is too cold to walk. You decide this might be a good time to switch into the Eat More, Exercise Less toggle. Get the picture?

DON'T LET HEC GET OUT OF CHECK EVEN IN MAINTENANCE

Even in maintenance, remember to watch your hunger level, your energy level, and your cravings. If you can't control cravings anymore, you need to modify the approach you have taken. If you've taken the wrong approach, your HEC will get out of check. One place where you can easily go off the rails is when you start to eat highly palatable foods again. Most of us have had the experience of going along fine with our diet, exercise, and healthy lifestyle. Then we decide to indulge a bit in a food we love, like pizza. And as soon as we do, it is as if we are taken over by some evil demon that is forcing us to eat everything in sight. All of a sudden, our cheat meal turns into a cheat week! Why?

There is an emerging understanding in research—mostly in animals, but quickly being confirmed in humans—that certain foods not only lead us to overeat at the current meal, but also cause cravings for more of those highly enjoyable foods later. Some have described this as being addicted to certain foods (usually highly palatable foods with a combination of starch, fat, and sugar or salt). While we don't yet have compelling evidence of food addiction, research is beginning to hint that there may be some truth to this notion.

A study published in March 2010 in the *International Journal of Obesity* showed this in rats. The animals were given their standard rat chow. Then they were divided up into different groups that had free access to either extra fat (HF), extra sugar (HS), or extra fat and sugar (HFHS).

If this experiment were done on humans, it would be as though you and your friends were separated into groups in which you ate a healthy diet plus had unlimited free access to bacon, cream cheese, and other high-fat items for those in the high-fat group. Or perhaps you were in the group that had access to cotton candy, Pixy Stix, Coca-Cola, and other high-sugar, no-fat items: the high-sugar group.

The HEC Check

Like in every phase, you have to adjust and tweak if something is going wrong and you're not burning fat or, worse, you're gaining it. If this is the case in this phase:

◎ Go back to the 3-2-1 or 4-2-2 approach.

◎ Do not try to eat less and exercise more for long, because it will likely make things worse.

◎ Avoid foods that combine starch and sugar or starch and fat—perhaps even the "healthy" ones like rice cakes or full-fat yogurt.

◎ Reduce your carbohydrate intake.

◎ Reduce your fat intake.

◎ Remember to focus on the diet inputs, *not* exercise, because compensating with exercise will often make things worse and is never the best approach to balancing the metabolism.

◎ If a slight decrease in carbs or fat doesn't work, then knock off a little more.

◎ The key to success is keeping your HEC in check and knowing your tolerance for the foods that cause you issues if you overdo them.

Or maybe you got to be in the high-fat and high-sugar group, which received the normal healthy diet plus cookies, cakes, pastries, ice cream, and other foods loaded with both fat and sugar, which you could eat freely: the high-fat and high-sugar group.

In the study, rats were essentially divided up like this. What do you think happened to them? Well, rats are like humans when it comes to food. If you give them all they can eat of enjoyable foods, they do what we do: eat more. They eat the normal rat chow and then chow down on the fat and/or sugar items. But also

The Protein Debate

The world of nutrition is funny. Back in the 1980s, we were told that fat would kill us. Then it was carbs we were urged to remove from our diet. And now there are some people out there telling us to banish protein from our diets forever. The question is: Why does everyone keep getting this wrong? Why is someone always coming up with a new food demon? Our opinion: Those making these proclamations have very strong biases toward their own ways of eating and are relying on the poorest forms of research to reach their conclusions. They're using population studies. It's fair to say this research can at times be useful if done well, and it most certainly is important work. But this type of research is not designed to prove anything. It at best shows correlations. It can't prove anything because there are so many variables to consider and everyone is so very different.

Let's use low-calorie alternative sweeteners as an example. If you did a population study to see who is using these products, the results would show that consumers who use them are mostly obese and overweight. At that point you might wrongly assume that these sweeteners are causing the obesity problem. In reality, however, that is wrong: They only correlate with it. The truth is that people who are obese and overweight are simply more likely to be on a diet and therefore to use these products. See how a population study can easily steer you to the wrong conclusion? There have been population studies showing that every single macronutrient—protein, fats, and carbs—will be the death of you. And this is the like us humans, the rat metabolism works like a thermostat and will ultimately adjust. And that is indeed what happened in all the groups except one. All three groups started out consuming much more food and those extra calories caused weight gain. But within a week or so, the rats in the high-fat group and the high-sugar group started to seem bored with the food and were able to self-regulate their food intake downward, lowering their calories and shutting off the hunger urge. But this natural adaptation did *not* occur in the group getting a combo of fat and sugar. That group continued gorging themselves as if they had turned into

primary reason we have been confused every third day by a new incorrect report from the media. When the data are tested in what is known as a randomized controlled trial, where, say, protein is added to replace carbs or fats, the message is clear: People lose more weight, have healthier blood values, and maintain their muscle tissue and strength. Several studies have looked at whether protein actually causes any of the purported side effects these biased writers and food zealots want you to believe it does. All those warnings about kidney and liver issues? Simply not true, and there is no evidence to suggest that it's a problem. In fact, the number one way to damage your liver and kidneys is to become diabetic, and that is more likely an issue of sugar, *not* protein.

There is no question that a plant-based diet is the healthiest. It is also our belief that you should eat whole, real foods whenever possible rather than protein shakes. But after doing this work for many years, we have found that a plan that is perfect but also impossible to do is in fact not a perfect plan. Therefore, there are many benefits to using convenient functional foods like protein powders. In addition, the proof is in the pudding. If your HEC is in check, you are losing fat, and your blood values are moving in a healthy direction, then it does not matter if you are living on nothing but jelly beans every day. If you are healthy, then that is the diet you should be following. The sooner the nutrition noisemakers grasp this concept, the better off we will all be.

gluttonous, food-addicted sloths. The researchers wrote that something about the high-fat and high-sugar diet was circumventing the normal reward and satiety centers of the brain.

A similar study in humans who had unlimited free access to highly palatable vending machine foods resulted in them eating 1,500 calories over their typical intake and gaining 5 pounds in just 7 days.

This effect seems so powerful in animal research and we have seen it so often in our clinic that we go to great lengths to warn our patients about these types of foods. This is why the 3-2-1 and 4-2-2 plates say "starch or fat." It is not that these foods are so bad in their own right; rather, it is that they almost always lead most of us to consume more and more of them.

 ## BE AWARE OF THE NEGATIVE SPIRAL: CHOOSE YOUR FOOD

Which foods are on our watch list, especially at this stage, when you might feel like the heavy lifting of weight loss is over? Foods high in a combination of any of the following:

◎ Salt   ◎ Sugar

◎ Fat   ◎ Starch

So these are foods containing both fat and sugar (like doughnuts), or sugar and salt (like yogurt-covered pretzels or caramel corn), or, most concerning, fat, sugar, and salt (like ice cream and desserts). Even foods containing fat and starch (like bagels and cream cheese, pizza, or bread with butter) can be an issue for some. These foods may seem to be the only things that will satisfy a craving or crush your hunger in the short run, but they typically make you crave more of those same foods later. This is why you want to do your best to avoid them whenever possible.

Eating some of these foods can make certain people end up in a negative spiral of cravings and eating large amounts of food and regaining weight. It also seems there may be a genetic component to this, so pay close attention to your individual reactions to these foods when choosing your cheat meal. If your cheat meal turns into a cheat week, then you will quickly know what the deal is and that you need to dial things back. Remember, the best way to help an unbalanced metabolism recover is to revert back to the full 3-2-1 or 4-2-2 approach.

Draw on all you've learned in this book to make sure you continue to seek balance. Keep your HEC always in check. That's your goal.

IT'S A PROCESS, ALWAYS CHANGING

In our experience, people prefer to be *looking* for something to do, rather than actually doing something. Translation: Oftentimes, even if we find something that works, we still feel the need to seek out something else. Maintenance is a process that needs to be practiced and mastered over time rather than a protocol that is followed for a short while and then abandoned for something else. That is the dieter's way of thinking, not the diet detective's. You will need to guard against this dieter's mentality in the maintenance phase. The path to mastery comes through practicing what you know again and again and avoiding the natural human tendency to try to find something else.

Think of it like learning to play a musical instrument or learning a new language. You continue to practice over and over again. You don't just learn to play the violin one day and then put it down; you keep at it. The process of body change is the same. Maintenance is an ongoing journey. The behaviors, the HEC check, the staying on track and balanced—all of this needs to be reinforced over and over and over so they become habits. A lot of what we've talked about in this book is biochemical, but there's a huge behavioral component too.

There's another important factor to consider in this phase: Your metabolism is constantly changing and adapting and reacting. It's never static. In women, for example, it changes fairly predictably every month according to the menstrual cycle. But there are many other factors that impact the metabolism more frequently and less predictably. So you've got to keep on top of it all the time.

What Could Change Your Metabolism Weeks, Months, or Years into Maintenance?

In the middle of your process, just as you're mastering being a diet detective, something could throw your system for a loop. There are many things that could impact the hormonal balance you've achieved.

- ⊚ Aging
- ⊚ Drugs
- ⊚ Illness
- ⊚ Menopause or andropause
- ⊚ Periods of overeating or under-eating

- ⊚ Periods of sleep deprivation
- ⊚ Pregnancy
- ⊚ Oral contraceptives
- ⊚ Overtraining or under-exercising
- ⊚ Short periods of increased stress

With your metabolism constantly in flux, you'll need to tap in to the skills you've learned, check your HEC, watch for changes in your body composition, and make sure you're always moving in the right direction. Learn to decipher the shifts. If you're struggling and can't figure it out, get to the doctor and get your laboratory evaluations done to make sure you're on track and getting healthier. We recommend getting blood labs done four times per year.

Metabolism Troubleshooting: Biofeedback Mechanisms

We've focused on hunger, energy, and cravings, but there are other elements to watch out for and assess to see if your metabolism is changing. They are:

- ⊚ Mood
- ⊚ Digestion

- ⊚ Exercise recovery
- ⊚ Sleep

Mood

Mood going out of balance can result from chronic stress, sleep deprivation, lack of exercise, or any number of life changes. Can we change our mood? Sure we can, and we have even seen these diet and lifestyle changes conquer clinical depression and anxiety when drugs were failing. Food, exercise, and sleep definitely impact your mood. Exercise is the number one way. Movement is a great antidepressant—probably the best one available without a doctor's prescription. This is where the benefits of traditional aerobic-based exercises shine. They are very good at elevating your mood. Walking gives many of those same benefits without the negative HEC effects. But for those susceptible to mood issues, completely cutting out traditional cardio may not be wise. We know from research that mood is best raised by moderate-intensity, long-duration exercises like jogging, biking, and running. So if these activities stabilize your mood, by all means do them.

Other Ways to Improve Your Mood

◎ Eating frequently can help; low blood sugar is associated with anxiety and depression.

◎ Make sure you get adequate sleep. Sleep deprivation is known to make us anxious, depressed, and crabby.

◎ Don't completely cut out starch if you have mood issues. Going too low can cause problems.

◎ Don't eat too much starch or sugar. Find the right balance for you.

◎ Getting in enough protein stabilizes blood sugar, and the amino acids that make up protein are the building blocks for all your brain chemicals.

◎ Cocoa and coffee can help you get focused and relaxed and lift depression.

◎ Herbal teas containing passionflower, lemon balm, chamomile, hops, valerian, and others can help calm anxiety.

Digestion

Whether it's the case at the start or it develops later, you might notice you're getting some digestive upset, which could reveal itself as gas, bloating, or an upset stomach. Your HEC could be in check and you could be burning fat, but it could still happen. And that usually means you'll gain weight. That's because the digestive tract is probably the most important of our metabolic organs. It is a major center of the nervous system, the hormone system, and the immune system. It is a window into your global metabolic function.

If your digestion is or starts to be disordered, then that's an indication of trouble ahead, which you'll eventually see as out-of-check HEC. If this is the case, start by assessing whether maybe you've developed a food allergy or sensitivity. Some typical food sensitivities include processed foods, grains, gluten, and dairy. If this is you, try our simple Digestive Restoration Program.

DIGESTIVE RESTORATION PROGRAM: THE 5R PROGRAM

This is a program you can use to restore balance to your digestive system. Remember, more than 50 percent of the immune system resides in the gut, so by correcting imbalances in the gut we can make effective changes in the immune system. And because the immune system overlaps with the nervous and hormonal systems, this is a great way to restore metabolic function. This program is the best way to help deal with gastrointestinal issues and is better than any detox program you could think of. It lasts for several weeks and works as follows.

Remove

The first step is to remove the cause of the inflammation in the gut. There are several different kinds of triggers for inflammation in the digestive tract. Food allergies or intolerances are the most common culprits.

To heal gut function and restore integrity to the digestive tract, elimination of these damaging triggers is your first priority. Botanical and nutritional approaches to stop or slow the inflammation are also available.

This entails reverting back to the 3-2-1 program, then adding a hypoallergenic diet to it, which means that you eliminate:

◎ Grains except for rice and quinoa (remember, corn is a grain)

◎ Dairy

◎ Nightshades (potato, tomato, eggplant, and all peppers)

◎ Beans and legumes (including peanuts)

◎ Eggs

◎ Soy

◎ Any other foods you feel you may be reacting to

That means you're doing 3-2-1 and eating animal protein, all vegetables except for nightshades, fruits, and nuts and seeds except for peanuts. Take all of the other foods out of your diet for 4 weeks, then challenge yourself with one of them every 4 days to see if any reactions come up. If you have a reaction, you should eliminate that food indefinitely. If you don't have a reaction, you can add that food back into your diet. This is super easy to do when following a 3-2-1 approach because instead of worrying about managing too many meals, you only have to worry about the last meal because the other two meals will be a hypoallergenic, dairy-free (no whey or casein), egg-free, and soy-free protein powder. It will make it easy for you to stick to the parameters and do the test best.

Replace

Following the removal of these substances from the digestive system, it is necessary to replace the body's natural defense against allergens, chemicals, and stress. The body uses digestive enzymes to break down substances for digestion and for protection. Adding extra digestive enzymes to boost the body's own supplies give the body time to heal. These digestive enzyme preparations can be found in the supplements aisle of your drugstore or health food store. You can find the one we use at our clinic at metaboliceffect.com/product /metabolicenzymes if you would like to see what a good digestive enzyme contains: lipase, amylase, protease, trypsin, chymotrypsin, and perhaps a small amount of betaine HCl.

Repopulate

The digestive system has many different healthy bacteria living in it. Normally these bacteria protect and communicate with the body and assist in digestion. If there are not enough of these healthy bacteria or there are too many of the wrong types, poor health results. In order to restore balance and health to the gut and the body, healthy bacteria are needed to repopulate the gut. These substances can also aid in fat loss by decreasing digestive efficiency. You can think of these friendly bacteria like that annoying friend who keeps stealing french fries off your plate: They can reduce your caloric intake. One 12-week study using a strain of good bacteria called *L. gasseri* resulted in a loss of 2 pounds and half an inch off the waist in some subjects without any change in diet or exercise. The research in this area is brand-new and evolving very fast. What we now know is that these gut bacteria are essential to metabolic function. We also know that the more biodiversity you have in your GI tract, the better. This means that having a lot of different types of organisms in your gut is better than having fewer. The frequent use of antibiotics may be a major disruptor of the delicate balance among the bacteria residing in our GI tracts. While yogurt and other products do contain bacteria, if you are really dealing with digestive upset, you will want to supplement with probiotics. If you would like to see the high-quality probiotic we use for patients in our clinic, please check our Web site.

Repair

Once the gut has all it needs in the form of enzymes and bacteria, nutrients and diet are used to repair any remaining damage. This is the most important part of the program, and one that is usually missed. In order for the GI tract to completely heal, this step is required. It will ensure that the digestive system returns to optimal function.

This stage includes adding compounds like glutamine and N-acetyl glucosamine (not the kind of glucosamine you take to help your joints) as well as healing herbs such as aloe and slippery elm. One great food that can go a long way toward healing the GI tract is sauerkraut (fermented cabbage). There are many great supplements you can purchase to aid in this. We use one in our clinic called GI Restore.

Be a diet detective with the 5R's as well. You may find you need to increase the length of time you use a gut restoration protocol depending on your system. Our colleague and partner at the Metabolic Effect clinic, Dr. Jillian Sarno Teta (Keoni's wife), is one of the premier integrative gastroenterologists in the country and has an excellent book on the subject called *Natural Solutions for Digestive Health*. We strongly suggest you read this work if digestive dysfunction is holding you back from your weight-loss goals.

Reintroduce

At the end of 4 weeks you will reintroduce the foods you eliminated to see if you are able to tolerate them or if they are an issue for your metabolism.

It is best to test foods you miss eating first. If you are reactive, this is a great reinforcing reminder of why you should continue to avoid the food. If you are not reactive, you get to add it back and enjoy a bit more variety.

It can take up to 4 days for a food reaction to develop. For this reason, you must reintroduce foods one at a time and wait 4 days between each food reintroduction. This helps isolate a reaction to any one food.

Be very careful in this stage. Test only one food at a time. For example, you would not want to reintroduce foods by eating a pizza, which contains wheat (gluten), dairy, and tomato (nightshades). Those are three potentially reactive foods. Instead, you would want to test them all individually. For example, you might test the wheat first. Wait 4 days, then challenge with dairy. Wait 4 more days, then experiment with tomato. This allows you to pinpoint exactly which foods are an issue for you.

If you do have any reactions, eliminate that food for 3 to 6 months before testing it again. There are many different reactions possible, but the most common food reactions include:

- Headaches
- Skin outbreaks, including rashes or acne
- Illness
- Joint pain
- Digestive upset
- Itchy skin
- Mood changes

One of the most amazing things we have seen in our clinical practice is the power of this 5R process to aid weight loss and heal many issues that conventional medicine struggles with, most notably autoimmune conditions.

DIET DETECTIVE: EXERCISE RECOVERY

In addition to keeping your eye on how your body's working and other forces impacting your maintenance, you need to continue to assess your workouts and how they make you feel. Your ability to perform well during exercise, and to recover adequately from it, is a great way to assess your metabolic balance. If you notice that workouts that used to be easier start becoming more difficult, this may signal that you are moving into the Eat Less, Exercise More trap. This is often a first warning sign in athletes who suffer from overtraining. If you are fueling your body correctly, you should notice slow improvements in your fitness. If you are not seeing this, then be aware that something is off. Soreness, aches, and pains resulting from exercise can help you assess things as well. It is normal and in fact beneficial to have soreness as a result of weight-training workouts. What is not normal is feeling sore constantly. If you are noticing that you are sore for much more than a few days, this may be a sign of inadequate recovery. This is often an issue with nutrition, such as taking in too few calories or carbs or inadequate protein. Soreness lasting several days is more frequent in beginners who have done very little exercise and are now becoming active. Once you are active, exercise soreness should not be chronic and should always resolve within a few days.

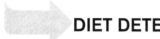 ## DIET DETECTIVE: SLEEP

If you can optimize your sleep, you will notice far less impact from stress. Sleep is a huge part of stress management. Remember: Rest and recovery are pieces of this puzzle, and sleep and stress management go hand in hand with both. Doing more rest and recovery during the week will aid you in getting a good night's sleep, which will in turn decrease your level of stress, which, as we have discussed, contributes to fat-burning weight loss.

It's also a chicken-and-egg scenario: As your metabolism regulates and heals and you lose weight, your sleep will improve. As you start to sleep better, you'll notice your metabolic function steadily improving.

Having said that, we are fully aware that if we could solve sleep management issues for everyone, we would be miracle workers. Everyone wants that formula. Dealing with insomnia is one of the most difficult clinical issues we confront. For our purposes, we want you to understand that nutrition and blood sugar balance are both parts of the sleep equation and that carbohydrates, protein, and fat play significant roles in your ability to fall asleep and stay asleep.

Sleep Hacking

◎ Difficulty falling asleep?

- You may be getting too few carbohydrates at night or not eating them close enough to bedtime.

◎ Waking up at 3:00 a.m.?

- You might not be getting enough fat and protein in your last meal of the day or you are eating too far ahead of bedtime.

We have found that simple adjustments have helped probably half of our patients fall asleep better and stay asleep longer. If you can get your sleep right, it has a significant impact on hormone balance.

What we can't adjust with diet, we can adjust with some behavioral tweaks. If you're plagued by sleep-lessness, consider:

- Installing blackout shades
- Moving your electronics away from your bed; some people find the electromagnetic radiation from their mobile devices impacts them.
- Playing white noise—visit the free site simplynoise.com.

Natural Sleep Aids

- Magnesium glycinate: Take 300 to 600 milligrams before bed
- GABA precursors such as Yogi's Bedtime Tea and the supplement GABA Calm (see metaboliceffect .com)

- Developing a pre-bedtime sleep routine by building in downtime for taking a hot bath, doing some light reading, staying away from bright screens, and not eating junk food
- Avoiding stimulants like caffeine during the day
- Avoiding alcohol as a sleep aid
- Making sure your sleep environment is cool (around 68°F is optimal)

If you're sleeping great, then your HEC will be more likely to be in check. If all of a sudden that changes and you start having sleep issues, your HEC will most certainly go out of check. If you do wake up at night, you may want to eat some carbs or carbs and fats, like a piece of banana and a spoonful of peanut butter, then try to get back to sleep as quickly as possible.

THE LOSE WEIGHT HERE RECAP

- The work doesn't end once you've settled into your desired weight. You have to keep assessing, investigating, and modifying to keep your HEC in check.
- You'll still use the 3-2-1 and 4-2-2 protocols you've learned. Most weeks you'll be in Weekend Warrior mode, doing 3-2-1 during the week and 4-2-2 on week-ends, incorporating a couple of cheat meals into the mix.

- You'll use your knowledge of the metabolic toggles to adjust through four different routines depending on where life takes you:
  - Eat Less, Exercise Less (ELEL)
  - Eat More, Exercise More (EMEM)
  - Eat More, Exercise Less (EMEL)
  - Eat Less, Exercise More (ELEM)

- You'll know how and when to toggle based on life circumstances, HEC changes, and all you've learned as a diet detective.

- Keep your eye on your mood, sleeping patterns, and digestion, as well as your exercise recovery time. These are extra pieces of biofeedback on your metabolic function.

- Most important, this is a lifestyle.

THE SCIENCE: *Weight and Aging*

Most of us do not realize that being overweight accelerates aging. In fact, any negative lifestyle habit, such as lack of sleep, poor nutrition, or being sedentary, puts one at more risk for chronic disease and weight gain. And chronic diseases like cardiovascular disease, type 2 diabetes, and most cancers accelerate the aging process by increasing the following:

1. **Chronic inflammation.** This is a cellular stress on the body usually triggered by excessive caloric consumption, high blood sugar, or increases in what are known as "reactive oxygen species." Think of these as molecules that cause you to rust internally.

2. **Glycation.** This is the result of sugar molecules—fructose and glucose, for example—binding tightly to protein or fat molecules, thereby rendering them useless to the body. Examples of glycation's presence in the body are cataracts, high blood pressure (hardening of the arteries), age spots, diabetic nerve damage, and LDL cholesterol plaques in the arteries. Think of this as forming particles that cause your body to caramelize and brown, much like the crispy sugar coating of a crème

brûlée. Once this occurs, the functioning of the cellular machinery is damaged.

3. **Improper methylation.** Methylation is the attachment of a methyl group (CH3) to other organic compounds. It acts as a switch that turns on and off various biochemical processes. Inappropriate methylation can turn genes off, like genes that reduce cancer risk, thereby increasing the likelihood of getting cancer. You can think of methylation as a sock you put on a foot to keep it warm and protected. Having socks with a bunch of holes in them is no good.

4. **Telomere shortening.** Telomeres are caps at the ends of chromosomes. They tell the body's "time," like a biological clock: The longer they are, the healthier and longer-lived you will be. Telomere shortening is primarily caused by cell division, aging, and chronic disease. You can think of a telomere like the plastic at the end of a shoelace—when it comes off, the strands of the shoelace can fray and shorten.

5. **Cellular debris.** This is the garbage—things like defective tau proteins, beta-amyloid, lipofuscin, and choles-terol plaques—that collects within the arteries. As the garbage increases, cell function decreases, ultimately leading to cell destruction. This is like junk mail piling up on your kitchen table; it serves no purpose and disrupts the use of your table.

As we age, our bodies become more and more unforgiving of our unhealthy lifestyle choices. This is due to many of the biochemical processes just mentioned. Even without any disease, we tend to naturally gain fat and lose muscle as we age. But is there a way we can stop or, at the very least, slow down the process of fat gain?

Many things are out of our control. Stressors like environmental pollutants can be minimized, but never eliminated. Also, the impact of environmental chemicals pales in comparison to the amount of damage our own bodies create internally when we make poor lifestyle choices. The great thing about bad habits is that we can change them by making and practicing new choices. And changing to more healthy habits can have an immediate positive change that you can feel.

So how do you know if your lifestyle habits are less than optimal and you are aging faster than you should? The most obvious way is to check your waistline with a tape measure. If your waistline is larger than your hips, you are overweight or obese and have already drastically accelerated your aging. The diagram below is a good guide to use in order to assess your waist-to-hip ratio. You can also use the diagram below to assess your health by checking your body mass index (BMI) and body fat percentage. Of the three measures (waist-to-hip ratio, BMI, and body fat percentage), a waist-to-hip assessment is probably the easiest to do. All it requires is measuring around your waist (the smallest circumference between the ribs and the belly button) and hips at their widest point. Once you have these measurements, you divide the waist measurement by your hip measurement to get the ratio. You have already learned how to use some of these measurements to understand the reshaping of your body, but the same points can be used to assess health. Achieving an hourglass or V shape is not possible when belly fat is elevated.

Another very useful measurement of your health and aging status is checking your blood pressure. In fact, high blood pressure is considered to be one of the most significant indicators of poor health and life expectancy. Most Americans have less than optimal blood pressure read-

WAIST CIRCUMFERENCE/BMI/BODY FAT %

◎ Waist > Hips = very high risk for disease and acceleration of aging

◎ BMI = mass in kilograms ÷ (height in m²) or weight in pounds ÷ (height in inches²) x 703

WAIST-TO-HIP RATIOS

Men	Women	Range
≤0.95	≤0.8	Optimal
0.96–1.0	0.81–0.85	Average
>1.0	>0.85	High Risk

BODY FAT % AND BMI

Men	Women	Range
10–14%, 20–24.9	18–22%, 20–24.9	Optimal
15–25%, 18.5–24.9	23–30%, 18.5–24.9	Average
>25%, >25	>30%, >25	High Risk

metaboliceffect.com

ings. Over time, high blood pressure damages your blood vessels and can lead to many issues, with heart attacks and strokes leading the way. And one of the most common causes of high blood pressure? Excess body fat is usually the culprit. Checking your blood pressure is very easy these days and does not require a visit to your doctor. You can check it at the drugstore or get a fancy home unit that works with your mobile phone. Measure it once a week. With a positive change in your lifestyle habits, your weight will come down, your blood pressure will fall, and the rate at which you are aging will slow.

The table below shows the 10-year risk of a cardiovascular (CV) event like a stroke or heart attack with increasing blood pressure for both women and men.

Probably the best objective way to measure how fast you are aging, and to get an assessment of where you are on the health continuum (with optimal health at one end and disease or death at the other), is by measuring the blood values in the diagram below every 3 to 6 months (or at least yearly). These labs are usually done on people who have already been diagnosed with certain diseases, but almost never on the average healthy person. We recommend that you find a physician who will run these labs for you, like an integrative or naturopathic physician. In our opinion, any doctor should be thrilled that you are proactively looking for ways to improve your health.

A fasting glucose measurement is always part of a conventional comprehensive metabolic profile (CMP). That is the

BLOOD PRESSURE (BP)

◎ Easy to check

◎ Chance of having heart attack or stroke increases dramatically as BP increases

BP Range (mm Hg)	% CV Risk Women	% CV Risk Men
Optimal <120/80	1.9	5.8
Normal 120/80– 130/85	2.8	7.6
High Normal 130/85– 140/90	4.4	10.1

metaboliceffect.com

Kurzwell, R. and Grossman, T. *Transcend*. Rodale 2009, pg. 198.

ANTIAGING BLOOD LABS

Labs	Conventional Range	Optimal Levels
Fasting glucose	65–99 mg/dL	65–85 mg/dL
Fasting insulin	2.6–24.9 µIU/mL	2–6 µIU/mL
Hemoglobin A1c	5–7%	4.3–4.7% or less without hypoglycemia
Homocysteine	6.1–15 µmol/L	<7 µmol/L
High-sensitivity C-reactive protein	<1.0– 3.0 mg/L	<1.0 mg/L
Serum 25-hydroxyvitamin D	30–100 ng/ml	50–100 ng/ml

metaboliceffect.com

test every doctor automatically does. The CMP includes many important measures of health status and should be done on at least an annual basis; however, the most important parameter for someone generally considered healthy is the fasting glucose value. Most overweight people have a fasting glucose reading that is high normal or above. It is also considered a snapshot of how fast you are aging. A good fasting glucose should be less than 85 milligrams per deciliter without having low blood sugar symptoms. As the name implies, a fasting glucose level is highly correlated with the amount of refined starches one eats, but it can also indicate stress reactions in the body, since stress hormones can elevate blood sugar.

Fasting insulin is a blood test that most conventional doctors will run only on diabetics, especially if they are insulin dependent. For the average person interested in fat loss and optimal aging, it is absolutely necessary to know. You should insist that your doctor run it. Insulin is a hormone secreted by the pancreas that moves blood sugar into your cells, where it can be burned for fuel or changed into fat for storage. High levels of insulin are positively correlated with high blood pressure. The higher your insulin level, the higher your blood pressure and the higher your risks of obesity, diabetes, Alzheimer's disease, cancer, and heart disease. Consumption of many dry starches, sweet carbohydrates, and starch and fat or sugar and fat combinations, as well as excessive calorie intake, raise your fasting insulin level.

Hemoglobin A1c (HbA1c), or glycosylated hemoglobin, is a measure of the amount of glycation occurring in hemoglobin, the oxygen-carrying proteins in your red blood cells. Since red blood cells live an average of 120 days, HbA1c gives an estimate of your average blood sugar over the previous 3 to 4 months. It is a great measure to assess how fast you are aging, especially in a healthy individual. The higher it is, the unhealthier the aging process in your body is. HbA1c is also closely tied to the amounts of starches and sweets you consume. The greater the consumption of these foods, the higher the HbA1c will be and the faster you will age.

Another very useful blood lab reflecting aging is something called the fructosamine test. Fructosamine is a compound that results from glycation between fructose or glucose and the protein albumin. Another way to think of this test is as a glycated albumin test. Like HbA1c, it gives you an estimate of blood sugar levels, but over a shorter time frame. Whereas HbA1c provides a view of the past 3 to 4 months, this test reflects only the previous 2 to 3 weeks.

Homocysteine is a marker of decreased methylation and inflammation. It is significantly influenced by dietary B-vitamin intake (especially natural forms of folate) as well as the amount of leafy green vegetables consumed. A veggie-based diet lowers levels of homocysteine.

High levels of homocysteine increase one's risks for stroke, dementia, cancer, and many other forms of chronic disease.

By far the best test to assess whole-body inflammation's impact on the cardiovascular system is high-sensitivity C-reactive protein (hs-CRP). CRP is synthesized by the liver in response to inflammatory chemical messengers released by immune and fat cells. The fatter one is, the more likely it is that hs-CRP levels will be high. The higher the hs-CRP level, the greater the risk of a heart attack. Health care providers usually run this test on individuals with known heart disease risk factors. But to be proactive, we suggest you get it done along with your routine labs.

One of the best lab values to know in order to help prevent almost all disease states is vitamin D. This is because it influences the body in so many ways. The test to ask for is called a serum 25-hydroxyvitamin D test, or 25(OH)D test. Vitamin D is protective against many types of cancer, autoimmune diseases, dementia, and bone diseases, especially osteoporosis. In the kidney, 25(OH)D (calcifediol) changes into the most active form of vitamin D (calcitriol). When supplementing with vitamin D, the most biologically active form to use is vitamin D_3 (cholecalciferol), which is converted in the liver to 25(OH)D. Optimal levels are between 50 and 100 nanograms per milliliter for most people.

For people interested in longevity and a high quality of life, knowing your blood values for these metrics can show you where you are on the health continuum and allow you to manipulate your lifestyle in appropriate ways. If you are overweight or obese, many of these metrics will be less than optimal. As you drop excess fat, you will see these metrics improve, and you will slow down the aging process. When one looks at the major factors that influence these metrics, it is difficult not to place most of the blame on excessively high intakes of refined starches, sweets, and starch, sugar, and fat food combinations, all of which make excessive caloric consumption inevitable.

Natalie

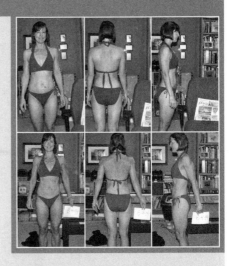

After giving birth to her third child, Natalie did what she thought was the right thing to do to get back into shape. She ate lots of protein and salad and did 1 to 2 hours a day of cardio. Her body didn't respond well. She was exhausted, not sleeping well, and had constant cravings. As soon as she read Metabolic Effect, she realized her hormones were out of whack. She made adjustments to her routine and her eating, ditching the intensive cardio for circuit training. Her body changed dramatically, her cravings no longer existed, and she was no longer, as she put it, "pigging out" in the middle of the night. She had renewed energy and confidence. After the birth of her fourth child, with her hormones in check, she bounced back immediately after the pregnancy.

When she decided to dive in a little deeper, she took on the Lose Weight Here plan. She learned more about her body's response to food and exercise and found her clothing fit better and was more comfortable. More important, she gained the experience of working with her body rather than fighting it, knowing what it needed in terms of nutrition and exercise. She's become toned, fit, and surprisingly didn't lose a pound despite a complete body transformation. She lost several inches and gained overall muscle mass. She liked the program so much that she became a trainer herself. She said she feels better now after giving birth four times than she did in her twenties.

Part III

Targeted Fat Loss

Michelle

Lose Weight Here changed Michelle. She was eating six meals a day working out 6 days a week. Once she (hesitantly) backed off the hard-core exercise, she learned to really tune in and listen to her body. She fed herself when she was hungry, not when she thought it was time to eat. Her entire mind-set shifted, and she started to really fine-tune the plan to meet her needs.

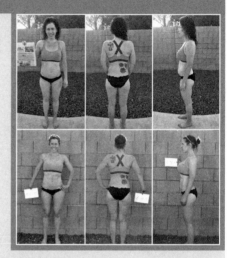

As she got deeper into the program, Michelle had an interesting revelation: Her body didn't react well to carbs, but it loved fat. Fat curbed her hunger and gave her energy. It helped her balance her cravings too. It's what challenged her so much in her earlier years—always being hungry and out of energy. It wasn't until Feed the Lean that she learned the secret.

Michelle didn't really want to move the scale, but she wanted to get rid of the little pooch she held on her stomach. She did, plus she lost an inch off her waist.

CHAPTER 8

SUPER BLAST:
Fat-Loss Foods

Food has become one of the most contentious issues in our society. It is like politics and religion in its ability to bring out people's biases. We, too, fell prey to that extremist thinking early on in our careers and found ourselves eagerly picking sides in the given nutrition debate of the moment, typically after reading a book on the subject.

We have literally been on every diet and been a member of almost every nutrition movement out there. We were low-fat followers in the late 1980s and early '90s. We then spent several years as militant vegetarians. Then, of course, we jumped on the low-carb Atkins craze—and on it went.

Finally, when we got out of medical school and started working with large groups of real people, we saw all of these nutritional practices had both an upside and a downside. Some people did fantastic as vegetarians and were the pictures of health. Some did very poorly, including myself (Jade)—Keoni and I are convinced my mostly vegetarian high-soy diet destroyed my thyroid. We have seen low-carb ketogenic diets work wonderfully for people and fail miserably for others. The Paleolithic approach to eating was a health-giving savior for some and a health disaster for others.

We have a favorite quote by Osho that says, "The less people know, the more stubbornly they know it." It took us a long time and many years of personal experience with thousands of people to realize that quote was so true of us in our younger years.

We now regard this food obsession and strong need to be on the "right team" in nutrition as one of the major sources of failure in health and fitness. We are not on Team Paleo or Team Vegetarian; rather, we are on both teams, and everything in between. There is only one rule in nutrition we now believe with all our hearts: Do what works for you.

That is why even in this chapter we are not giving you defined, strict meal plans, and we are not going to tell you to eat only certain foods and to always avoid others. As you have learned, that detective work is up to you. You must find through your own trial and error, using the AIM process (assess, investigate, and modify) that we have taught you, the plan that works for you. What we are going to help you understand now are the specific types of foods we have found are most successful for the vast majority of people. We call these fat-loss foods.

FAT-LOSS FOODS

Despite what you have been told, there is no such thing as food that has magical fat-burning properties. Anytime you eat anything, you will slow down fat burning. Why? Because the body now has other resources to burn instead. All this talk in the nutrition world about speeding up your metabolism with certain foods is a false statement.

Like many things, there is a speck of truth to it. Eating too little, as you have learned, certainly can cause metabolic compensation. And every single time you eat, the body needs to use energy to digest that food. This is called the thermogenic effect of eating. But the fact remains that when you eat, you take in calories that your body will burn instead of fat.

So what then is a *fat-burning* or a *fat-loss* food? It is simply a food that when eaten reduces hunger in the moment and causes lasting hunger suppression. It also balances energy and reduces the chance of metabolic compensation from dieting. In other words, fat-loss foods keep your hunger-energy-cravings (HEC) in check and make it far less likely you will—or can—overeat.

Now here is the tricky thing about fat-loss foods: They can be different for different people. For some, a bowl of oatmeal in the morning fills them up and keeps cravings at bay for the next 4 to 6 hours. For others, that same bowl of oatmeal may not suppress hunger and may trigger cravings and fat gain.

This is why meal plans, recipes, and the strictly defined guidelines of your average diet book almost always fail miserably. It is also the reason we refuse to allow you to fall into that trap and will tell you far less of this stuff than you likely have ever read in a diet book. This might make things harder on you in the short run, but it will eventually be the very thing that finally frees you from the diet trap.

The trick is to get in tune with how food impacts you. And the good news is that research has shown there is plenty of overlap from person to person; in other words, there are certain foods that seem to balance HEC and result in effortless calorie reduction for most people.

These foods are rich in protein, fiber, and water and deficient in starch and fat. Starchy foods and fatty foods can be very healthy, and many are also fat-loss foods, but there is far less room for error with these foods since people have various responses to them. For example, one person who eats bacon and eggs for breakfast can be healthy because it balances HEC and effortlessly results in weight loss; another person can eat that meal and end up starving later, resulting in binging the rest of the day.

There are also foods that tend to be detrimental for almost all people. These are foods that combine fat and starch/sugar or salt, or highly processed foods devoid of water.

So when it comes to figuring out your own fat-loss formula, start by eating as many foods as possible from the green list that follows. These are those protein-, fiber-, and water-rich foods that are lower in fat and starch. Next, determine which of the yellow group you can eat freely and which you will need to regulate. Finally, eat the red foods sparingly, infrequently, or never, depending on your individual tolerance. The green, yellow, and red designations are easy to remember: Green means go, yellow means proceed with caution, and red means stop.

This is how it works: The 3-2-1 and 4-2-2 plans provide a super-simplistic structure, and we advise you follow those protocols without deviation in the beginning. As you progress, experiment with how much of the green, yellow, and red foods you can include.

How Foods Affect HEC and Fat Storage

 Line one depicts typical reactions   Line two depicts individual reactions

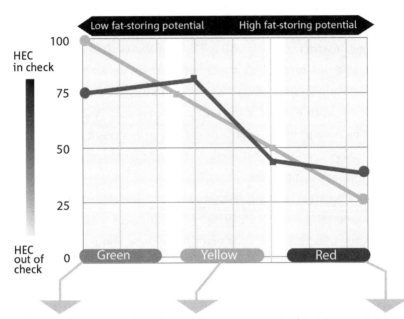

Low fat-storing potential   High fat-storing potential

HEC in check

100

75

50

25

HEC out of check   0

Green   Yellow   Red

Green (eat unlimited)

Protein: chicken, turkey, wild fowl, game meats, most fish, bison, lean ground beef, shellfish, lean cuts of pork, egg whites, and protein powders

Nonstarchy high-fiber veggies: kale, collards, Brussels sprouts, broccoli, cabbage, cauliflower, spinach, lettuce, salad greens, tomato, jicama, asparagus, green beans, cucumber, celery, peppers, carrots, radish, zucchini, squashes, pumpkin

High-water, low-sugar fruits: berries, apples, pears, citrus fruits

Yellow (eat to tolerance)

Fatty meats: lamb, fatty cuts of beef, fatty cuts of pork, fatty fish like salmon

Vegetable fats: avocado, olives, olive oil, coconut oil, vegetable oils, nuts and seeds, peanuts

Lower-fiber, high-sugar fruits: banana, melons, cherries, pineapples, mango, kiwi

Starchy low-fiber veggies: potatoes, corn, peas, sweet potatoes

Wet starches: potatoes, corn, peas, sweet potatoes, rice, quinoa, oats, cream of rice, beans and legumes

Dairy foods: milk, yogurt, butter, cheese

Whole eggs

Red (eat rarely if ever)

Dry starches: pasta, bread, crackers, pretzels, chips, rice cakes, cereals

Junk foods: cookies, cakes, candy, sweets, soda, etc.

Let's revisit the chart we introduced to you in Chapter 6.

The Green Foods

These are the most common fat-loss foods for the majority of people. Let's choose two items from this list: a grilled chicken breast and a cup of broccoli. For comparison, let's choose a common food from the red list: a "healthy" breakfast cereal—you know, something an MD or nutritionist might tell you to eat, like Kashi GoLean.

Now let's calculate the calories for 5 servings of each. Kashi GoLean Crunch!: 5 servings (5 cups) = 950 calories (per calorieking.com); 5 boneless, skinless chicken breasts (6 ounces each) = 936 calories; 5 cups of broccoli = 273 calories.

You could eat 5 chicken breasts and 5 cups of broccoli and have eaten only about 250 calories more than with 5 cups of Kashi. Think about the amount of food that is. Eating 5 cups of cereal would be relatively easy to do in a day; in fact, many people eat close to this amount every morning. Now consider the chore it would be to eat 5 chicken breasts and 5 cups of broccoli. The average person would be hard-pressed to eat that over an entire day, let alone in one meal. And which of these two would balance HEC, provide more nutrition, and be more likely to help you burn fat and gain muscle?

We hope this illustrates for you what we mean by fat-loss foods.

The Yellow Foods

Some of the foods in the yellow list are among the best hunger-suppressing foods on the planet. For example, the much-maligned potato is what we call a *wet starch*. Wet starches can be extremely satiating. In fact, when scientists studied the foods that are most satisfying, the potato beat out almost every single food.

So are we saying a potato is a fat-loss food? Yes! For many people it absolutely is. Including a wet starch with dinner may be the very thing that takes away the hunger and the craving for that pint of ice cream later.

Other wet starches include beans, rice, oats, corn, peas, and sweet potatoes. As long as you don't go adding a bunch of fat to these foods—which, unfortunately, most people do—they can certainly be healthy fat-loss foods for many people. But for others they can also easily be overdone, which is why they are in the yellow group. You will need to find your natural tolerance for these foods.

You will notice wet starches are used in both the 3-2-1 and 4-2-2 plans. In the 3-2-1, you eat them once per day, at night. In the 4-2-2, you eat them at two of your four meals, preferably in the hours after a workout. During both stages you tweak to find your tolerance.

You will also find all of your high-fat foods in the yellow group. Fat, like starch, is something you will need to determine your individual tolerance for. Be a detective instead of a dieter, and separate fat and protein. For example, eat all the low-fat chicken or bison meat you want, but avoid a fatty steak. This detective work will make your meal plan easier to follow.

A good rule of thumb when the green foods aren't filling you up is to add fat to your meals first. First, try doing so in the form of vegetable fats—things like avocados, coconut oil, olive oil, and nuts and seeds—or by adding a homemade Caesar dressing made with egg yolks. This will help you more thoroughly understand your reaction to fats and hit your HEC sweet spot.

You will also see dairy foods in this category. Dairy can be exceedingly healthy and fat-loss friendly for many people, but for others it can produce excessive insulin and result in overeating. Dairy often comes with sugar (lactose) in addition to fat. As with fats, it's best to experiment with whether low-fat or high-fat dairy foods are more appropriate for your HEC and fat-loss goals.

Certainly don't avoid dairy just because you heard it was bad. But don't make the mistake of eating it freely just because you heard it was good. The only way to know if it is a fat-loss food or a fat-storing food for you is to assess and investigate its effects on your metabolism.

And remember: We are making a distinction here between what is a healthy food versus what is a fat-loss food. A food can have plenty of positive nutritional elements to it, but if you remain overweight while you are eating it, it is not optimizing your health.

The Red Foods

These are the foods almost everyone will struggle with. This is not to say there won't be some who thrive on these foods. However, if they exist, they are in the minority. These foods can be enjoyed in limited amounts and occasionally, but this class of food is the most dangerous to play with.

This group actually contains three classes of foods: foods high in dry starch, foods high in sugar, and foods that combine starch or sugar and fat. This is also the group we put all forms of alcohol in. The reason these foods can be so detrimental can be seen in our earlier comparison between five servings of cereal and five each of chicken and broccoli. Dry starches like cereal, pasta, and bread are not very filling and have high calorie density: They contain a lot of calories in proportion to the amount you are eating. If you have ever measured out an actual serving of cereal or pasta and placed it in a bowl, you know exactly what we mean. It's a tiny amount.

There may be some confusion at this point because if you are like many people, you have (wrongly) been taught that these dry starches, especially whole grains, are the ones with the most fiber. And of course, as we have stated, fiber is good. This is another area where you need to be a little savvier in your nutrition knowledge. It is absolutely true that many dry whole grain starches have more total fiber compared to some vegetables, fruits, and wet starches. The problem is that the body works in relative proportions, not total amounts. In other words, it is far more important to know how much starch there is compared to fiber and water. You want the starch-to-fiber ratio to be more in favor of fiber than starch. Whole grains may have more total fiber, but they have far greater amounts of starch and come without the water benefit. The illustration below helps explain this concept.

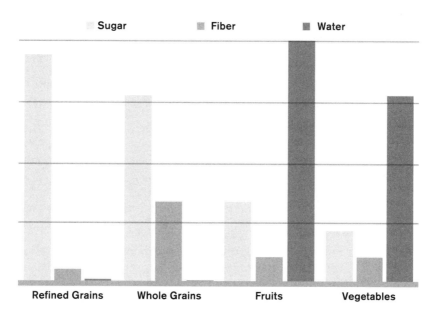

When fat is added to starch or sugar, these foods not only become calorically dense, but also may negatively impact your biochemistry by increasing food intake during the current meal and causing cravings for high-calorie foods at future meals.

Animal studies show these foods have a hedonistic effect, disrupting regulation of the hunger and craving centers in the animals' brains. These foods might be addictive, so eliminating them from the diet is often one of the most powerful changes you can make. In our experience, it takes a few weeks to break free of their spell, but it can literally release some people from a lifetime of food struggles.

Again, these foods are not horribly detrimental for every person, but given their effects on caloric intake and brain chemistry, it is best to limit them or avoid them completely. These foods include things like cakes, cookies, and pastries, but can also include pasta with cream sauce, pizza, bagels with cream cheese, french fries, and burgers. Ironically, while the potato can be a great fat-loss food when eaten in its natural form, in Western society it is almost never eaten this way, instead generally being served loaded with fat and salt.

STRESS AND FAT GAIN

Weight loss is about more than just calories. If it were as simple as calories, the obesity problem would be much easier to solve. There are other factors impacting the battle against weight: chiefly, sleep deprivation and chronic stress. Both negatively impact fat loss even though they are, in fact, calorie free. You can't eat them, yet they impact whether we store fat or burn it. They also dramatically impact our hunger, motivation to work out, and cravings. So while it is true that excessive calories cause weight gain, it is shortsighted to pretend that other factors don't have an impact.

The Body Is a Highly Complex Biochemical Machine

There is nothing more ignorant and judgmental, in our opinion, than assuming that anyone who does not get results from making changes to their diet and exercise regimen is not "following the rules." Or that those who are unable to control their eating are simply overeaters who don't work out and lack willpower, and should be berated.

The truth, as you have learned by now, is that when you start to assess all that actually makes us fat, the situation is more complex than we think. "Eat less, exercise more" is not the answer. In fact, fat gain and weight loss are both multifactorial and individualized—they involve understanding genetics, one's unique metabolic expression, psychological factors, and even personal preferences. But there do appear to be some overarching themes.

The Fat-Gain Formula

Want to know what the fat-gain formula is? (F + S) × St = Fat Gain. That is, high fat (F) plus high sugar (S) multiplied by stress (St) is the recipe for fat gain. This of course is an overly simple explanation, but it is a very useful model for understanding fat gain. Sure, you can get fat overeating anything; on that fact we agree. But it is virtually impossible for any person who gorges on chicken and greens to do so. It just won't happen.

A diet high in both fat and sugar has been shown in mammals to completely disrupt the normal metabolic regulation that occurs with either a high-fat or a high-sugar diet. So not only is it a higher-calorie diet, it also seems to assure that we continue to crave high-fat, high-sugar foods in the future. The combination of these two items alters brain chemistry in a way that disrupts your natural ability to regulate your caloric intake. The bottom line: Fat plus sugar will sabotage your willpower.

Here is how it works. You have a control center for appetite in your brain that resides in a gland called the hypothalamus. There are chemicals that stimulate appetite, called neuropeptide Y (NPY) and agouti-related peptide (AGRP), and there is one that suppresses food intake, called proopiomelano-cortin (POMC).

Think of NPY and AGRP as gas pedals: They make us hungry and make us eat. POMC, on the other hand, is the brake on this process. (If you are wondering how hunger hormones like ghrelin and leptin figure into this, it's that their signaling impacts the release of NPY, AGRP, and POMC.)

Two diets containing the same number of calories can impact these hunger-regulation chemicals differently. Fat and sugar in combination seems to "short-circuit" the hunger centers, resulting in a constant desire for food.

Remember the rat study we presented to you earlier in the book—the one where the rats eating sugar and fat together got fat? The same thing happens to humans. There's a hormonal explanation for this. The researchers noticed that the negative effects of the high-fat, high-sugar group were generated by hormonal signaling from the GI tract. Something about the high-fat, high-sugar diet that was communicated to the brain by the gut disrupted normal, healthy responses to eating.

A high-fat diet that has the same number of calories as a high-fat, high-sugar diet has a very different impact on metabolism. Your metabolism adapts to the extra calories in a high-fat diet by decreasing your appetite so that after a few weeks your caloric intake is no longer as high. This explains why studies on the high-fat Atkins diet usually show a lower caloric intake over time.

The combination of high fat and high sugar creates the exact opposite changes in the hunger-signaling molecules in the brain, resulting in ongoing, insatiable hunger. (Ironically, this is almost exactly the same pattern of changes seen in starvation.)

We can see that high-fat, high-sugar foods are not just simply higher in calories, but also alter our bodies' ability to regulate and suppress hunger, causing hyperphagia (the fancy medical term for continuous eating). And when we add chronic stress to this, we create the perfect fat-storing atomic bomb; more on this coming up next.

The Cherry on Top

Let's go back to the fat-storing formula for a second: $(F + S) \times St$, fat plus sugar multiplied by stress. Stress, it turns out, is the cherry on the top of this fat-storing sundae.

If you are a savvy fat-loss lifestyler or fitness professional, when you think about stress, you think about cortisol. And if you are really savvy, you will also think catecholamines. Really, *really* savvy? You will think of one more hormone: NPY. Remember that one? NPY is involved with hunger signaling, but it is also released from the sympathetic nervous system during times of stress.

When you are under acute stress, you release more catecholamines and cortisol; when you are under chronic stress, you release more NPY. And unlike catecholamines and cortisol, which are mainly catabolic hormones (meaning that they burn fat), NPY makes you gain fat. When NPY is released in large amounts, it causes fat cells to go from immature, baby fat cells to full-grown, mature fat cells. In addition, cortisol makes the body more responsive to NPY—in other words, while NPY alone makes fat cells grow, adding cortisol to the mix makes it more efficient at it.

Confused? Let's review it again: Chronic, continuous stress releases a unique mix of NPY and cortisol. But unlike when cortisol combines with catecholamines (in moments of short-term stress), which helps us burn fat, when cortisol combines with NPY (as happens with chronic stress), it increases fat-cell growth.

Another interesting aside about some of these studies on rodents: When you feed mice high amounts of fat and sugar, obesity is not guaranteed. But add stress on top and *boom*—you can induce obesity very easily.

One final note on your body's response to stress: Standard low-calorie diets can increase your levels of cortisol and perceived psychological stress, and some researchers believe this is one of the key reasons they fail.

CARB CONFUSION

Carbs are a hot topic of discussion for us. Many of our patients are initially obsessed with their impact, mostly because of the information overload regarding it. But eliminating carbs completely isn't the answer: Manipulating your intake of them and noting how they impact your body is. So don't ask yourself *if* you should eat carbs; ask yourself *how much* you should eat and *when*.

Carbs You Want to Eat for Fat Loss

Eat all the carbs from the green list of foods in unlimited fashion. These are primarily all the nonstarchy vegetables and low-sugar fruits—things like berries, apples, pears, and citrus. In addition, find your tolerance for the sweeter fruits and the wet starches. Remember to include the skin when eating potatoes, and never add fat to them. Many people who have eliminated carbs and experienced low energy and cravings as a result will notice amazing changes if they add wet starches back in. Oats, beans, rice, and quinoa, among others, can have amazing benefits on HEC and get you moving in the right direction. Don't let the carb nazis convince you to avoid something that might be beneficial. These foods can certainly play a great role in your fat-loss journey. If you are still skeptical, just look at the amount of wet starch that people in Asian countries tend to consume. They generally eat much more rice than we do in the Western world, yet they remain slimmer. What they also do—at least those eating traditionally—is eat plenty of produce and avoid adding excessive fat and salt to their starch.

The Carb Tipping Point

When you think about your tolerance for the starchy and sweet foods, it is helpful to use a tool we call the carbohydrate tipping point. This is the greatest amount of starchy and sweet foods you can eat that stabilizes HEC, gives you great performance in the gym, and does not slow fat loss or increase fat gain. This is different for all of us, and there is no greater use of your time as a diet detective than to solve this equation for yourself.

There are several aspects to this concept.

◎ Carbohydrate amount

◎ Carbohydrate type

◎ Carbohydrate timing

The *carbohydrate amount* is self-explanatory. You learned about this when we introduced you to the detective tool we call AIM. You simply start your process following the 3-2-1 or 4-2-2 structure we gave you, then tweak and adjust depending on your results. This may involve raising or lowering the amount of carbs by several bites or grams.

The *carbohydrate type* is a little trickier to work with. You just learned about all the different types of carbs: There are the nonstarchy veggies; the high-water, low-sugar fruits; the sweeter fruits; and the wet and dry starches. Eat the majority of your carbs in the form of veggies and less-sweet fruits, adding the other types as needed to balance HEC and burn fat.

One other aspect of carb type is important: allergy potential. You want to focus on the low-allergy-producing carbs, or what are known as "hypoallergenic carbs." These are low in chemicals that irritate the gut or cause immune reactions in the body. You may have heard that some people (but certainly not all, as the nutrition alarmists would have you believe) can have immune system reactions to gluten, which is present in many grains, especially wheat. Other carbs have high amounts of lectins and saponins, which can irritate the lining of the gut and cause gastrointestinal issues. These include grains, beans/legumes, and white potatoes. If you find you are sensitive to these carbs, choose veggies, fruits, sweet potatoes, rice, and quinoa instead. These are the least likely starches to cause issues.

Finally, *carbohydrate timing* is critical as well, so let's discuss that now.

Carb Timing Strategies

As they say, timing is everything. Here are a few strategies that might work for you. If you already employ one and it's working, don't be a research chaser. Stick with your routine.

Eating All Carbs Postworkout

Carbohydrates are a major stimulator of the muscle-building and fat-storing hormone insulin. After a workout is a great time to include carbs because exercise is an insulin mimicker. Just the act of contracting your muscles increases the number of glucose receptors on muscle cells. This is the same thing insulin does. So eating most of your starch after a workout allows for increased glucose uptake by muscles, which increases glycogen storage and muscle protein synthesis without much insulin. This accentuates the muscle-building impact of insulin and deemphasizes its fat-storing effects. Translation: It's the best of all worlds. Do keep in mind, though, that overloading on carbs postworkout immediately slows down fat burning.

Eating All Carbs in the Morning

Insulin sensitivity is highest in the morning, after your overnight fast, and lowest in the evening, after a full day of meals. This means that generally, there is less negative impact from eating starch in the morning compared with the evening. This morning approach might also cause some adjustments to your leptin curve, making it peak in the early evening instead of the middle of the night, which can have benefits in reducing hunger in the evening. If you find you are ravenous at night, first increase your protein intake. If that doesn't work, try this approach with your carbs. The morning strategy works well if you prefer a morning workout or if you're dragging during the day. It also works if you wake up craving pastries and coffee.

Eating Carbs When You Crave Them

If there is a particular time of the day you tend to crave starchy foods, there are two strategies to try. The first is to have your carbohydrates before that time—to beat the craving, essentially. For example, let's say you crave sweets or bread at 3:00 p.m. almost every afternoon. Ask yourself about your meal at lunch: Did you skip carbs or overload on them? This will tell you a lot about an approach that can work for you. Perhaps you need to trade in the gigantic burrito for a salad at lunch. Or perhaps you want to add a bit of starch to your tossed salad and chicken breast. Or maybe you want to save your daily carb allotment for that late afternoon snack so you can relax and attack the craving head-on.

Eating Carbs at Night

Carbohydrate intake is believed to trigger the release of serotonin, a relaxing brain chemical that can aid sleep, in the brain, though the discussion on this topic has sparked some controversy. Essentially, insulin pushes most other amino acids into the tissues, leaving tryptophan with less competition to cross the blood-brain barrier and raising serotonin in the process.

Eating starches at night can also lower cortisol and catecholamine levels, which can be elevated at night in people who experience insomnia. This strategy also works well for those who work out in the evening and/or crave starch at night. It might also help curb cravings the next morning.

Fine-Tuning Your Strategy

These strategies are not one-size-fits-all, and any expert who tells you otherwise is wrong. If you're at this stage and want to tweak your approach to eating carbs further, consider the following.

◎ Reducing your overall starch intake

◎ Eating starches only at specific times of the day

◎ Limiting starchy carbohydrates to 20 to 30 bites per day. We consider a bite to be 1 level tablespoon or about 5 grams of carbs, so this is 100 to 150 grams per day. We like using the number of bites because adjusting it to find your sweet spot is easier than changing a weight or measurement.

Also consider your habits.

1. Do you work out at night or have difficulty sleeping? Do you crave starch, salt, and/or sweets in the evening? Find yourself ravenously hungry in the morning? **If so, save your entire daily carb intake for the evening.** If you notice you sleep better and your hunger, energy, and cravings are better controlled the next day, and at the end of the week you see improvement in your body composition, you have moved one step closer to your metabolic formula.

2. Do you work out in the morning before eating? Crave coffee and pastries for breakfast? Notice low energy all day if you don't have morning carbs? Find yourself insatiably hungry at night? **Then eat all your carbs in the morning** and skip them the rest of the day.

3. Don't feel hungry for most of the day, or until after lunch? Have high energy despite not eating? Tend to hold on to your muscle mass? Get sick and tired of worrying about preparing meals for the day and stressing about what to eat? Able to go the whole day without food and still eat sensibly at night? **Consider fasting the entire day and eating only one big meal (including your carbs) in the evening.**

4. Feel low energy when you don't eat? Feel foggy-headed and can't think clearly unless you have carbs? Are you insulin resistant and prone to "feeling" hypoglycemic? Overweight or obese? New to the fat-loss lifestyle? **You will likely be better off eating small, frequent meals, with each meal containing a small amount of carbs (5 to 10 bites).** These meals should also contain a good portion of protein.

5. Have difficulty gaining muscle? Train intensely with weights? Having difficulty recovering from exercise? Are you an athlete with performance goals? **Then eat carbs postworkout as well.** Consider having 30 to 50 grams of whey protein and a large banana. It may give you an insulin kick at just the right time to take your fat-burning, muscle-building game to the next level.

Eating Frequency

Eating four to six meals a day is a weight-loss strategy, not a fat-loss one. What we mean by that is that weight loss is about one-size-fits-all "rules," whereas fat loss is about individualized adjustments. We don't adhere to these rules. Your eating frequency should be based on whether your HEC is in check. Remember: Body change is both art and science. The art of the process lies in knowing your own metabolic expression, psychological sensitivities, and personal preferences. Your friend may be able to skip breakfast, have a sensible lunch, and come home for dinner without cravings or insatiable hunger. You, on the other hand, may not be able to do this. You need to spend time finding your own personal approach that delivers results. After first adopting the Lose Weight Here lifestyle, many people will need to move toward eating more, rather than less, frequently. This approach is necessary for them because the compensatory reactions of their bodies are strong and relentless; hunger, energy fluctuations, and cravings are impossible to control for long on willpower alone. This may seem like a confusing statement in light of the 3-2-1 protocol, but it shouldn't be. At this point, you should be well acquainted with the idea of structured flexibility. You cannot expect your metabolism and needs to adhere exactly to what we laid out. If you find the 3-2-1 protocol simply does not stabilize your HEC unless you snack, then snack. Just make sure you measure the results to see if it works for you. What to snack on? The green foods, of course, are the best.

THE FASTING FIXATION

Fasting is a popular topic when discussing health and weight loss, and because of that, we feel it is important for you to consider it in your detective work. It can certainly be a valuable lifestyle strategy for fat loss, but you should understand all the considerations if you are going to explore whether it is right for you. We have many discussions with patients who want to know if fasting works as a tool for weight loss. Like any clues we seek as diet detectives, if something works well for you, we're not going to tell you to stop. Everyone is different psychologically and physically and in terms of lifestyle. And we believe there can be incredible benefits to fasting for your health. Whether or not it will result in sustained fat loss depends on you. The risk with fasting: It has enormous potential to backfire on you, so you need to know how to use it intelligently. Can fasting be incorporated into your healthy lifestyle, or will it result in metabolic compensation and yo-yo weight regain? Our answer: We have seen many people do wonderfully with it; we have seen many more crash and burn. There is nothing wrong with trying it, just do it with the mind-set of a detective, not a dieter. Gather information along the way to see if it is a good fit for you, and don't be afraid to adjust to fit your needs. We have observed that it is not the best approach for beginners, but it can be a great strategy for those who are further along in their fat-loss journey. Remember, there are three ways to tell if a strategy is working for you: 1) it keeps HEC in check; 2) it is moving you toward the hourglass or V-shape body type; and 3) it is optimizing your blood laboratory markers.

Can fasting be incorporated into your healthy lifestyle, or will it result in metabolic compensation and yo-yo weight regain? Our answer: There is nothing wrong with trying it, just do it with the mind-set of a detective, not a dieter. Gather information along the way to see if it is a good fit for you, and don't be afraid to adjust to fit your needs.

Fasting Risks for Some

- ◎ Constant hunger
- ◎ All-day cravings
- ◎ Overeating after a day of fasting, which we call a continuous meal
- ◎ No libido
- ◎ Tired, but wired

Fasting Benefits for Some

- ◎ Decreased body fat
- ◎ Greater energy
- ◎ Reduced hungry
- ◎ Fitness and strength

Fast or Fiction: Misconceptions about Fasting

Fasting and Blood Sugar

The people who say you should never skip meals make the point that doing so can lower blood sugar and lead to cravings later. Those who advocate fasting point to studies showing that blood sugar numbers remain stable despite clinical signs of hypoglycemia (low blood sugar). This is where nuance and shades of gray come in. The idea that all people are going to have a drop in blood sugar and go on a cheesecake binge if they skip a meal or fast is untrue. Many people skip meals every single day and are able to achieve lean, healthy bodies, and do so while keeping HEC in check. The same goes for people who eat more than three times per day. They, too, can attain and maintain very lean and healthy physiques with this approach. The trick is to discover which eating strategy is best for you: Should you eat small, frequent meals or only one or two meals per day while fasting the rest of the time?

> One person's fat-loss plan is another person's formula for being fat.

Part of this discovery requires looking past the rhetoric on both sides. Nothing is as simple as it seems, and as a diet detective you should embrace this complexity. Take the discussion about blood sugar, for instance. Assumptions that skipping meals or fasting is the solution for everyone and that the body is able to access blood sugar simply because its level is normal are wrong. These beliefs show a misunderstanding of insulin resistance, a condition present to some degree in almost all overweight and obese individuals. Those who are insulin resistant suffer from cellular hypoglycemia, or low sugar levels within cells. Think of a diabetic: Their cells can be deprived of glucose even when they have blood sugar levels many times above normal. While the brain does not require insulin to access blood sugar, insulin signaling in the brain is heavily involved in blood sugar regulation throughout the body. By the same token, a lack of sugar in any cell or tissue that needs it will result in alarm bells that ultimately reach the brain and force it to respond. This is why you see such severe hypoglycemic effects in some people even when their blood sugar is normal or even high. It is not "all in their head," as is sometimes suggested.

Fasting can cause similar blood sugar regulation issues and lead to compensatory eating later despite normal blood sugar levels. Some people are

Don't Seek the Expedient Solution

Just because a solution seems the most expedient does not mean it actually is. Sometimes slow and steady is far better than speedy and reckless. The fastest way to lower your insulin level might seem like fasting or skipping meals, but in an emergency, running for the exit as fast as you can usually causes more harm, not less. An organized, levelheaded approach often works best here. In the context of balancing blood sugar, this may mean eating frequent small meals having adequate protein content—the same diet doctors prescribe for true hypoglycemics.

more susceptible to this than others. This is why paying attention to HEC is so critical. It tells you immediately whether fasting is balancing your hormonal metabolism or disrupting it. The types of people who have their HEC thrown out of whack by fasting are often the worst possible candidates for this approach.

Fasting in Context

It is also important to not examine fasting in isolation. A person training with weights who also fasts is very different from a fasting person who is not weight training. Many of the negative effects of fasting come from not understanding how to properly pair it with training.

Fasting for 16 to 24 hours day after day while working a stressful job and engaging in high-intensity metabolic conditioning or cardiovascular workouts several times a week is not a great solution for the vast majority of people. This is an extreme version of eating less and exercising more. However, pairing fasting days with relaxation days and no-exercise days and then eating normally on training days is entirely different. The latter approach is much like the 3-2-1 and 4-2-2 protocols you have learned in this book.

It is important in all discussions of health and fitness to look at the big picture, which is why focusing only on what the research says is not always wise. Strictly focusing on research can blind you to the multifactorial nature of individual lifestyles and the metabolic expressions and stress susceptibilities of different people. That is why your best approach is always the one that feels right for you.

Ready to Fast?

◎ Your metabolism is balanced.

◎ You successfully completed the Eat Less, Exercise Less (ELEL) and Eat More, Exercise More (EMEM) programs and are at your ideal weight.

◎ You can go for long periods without food and then eat a normal fat-loss-friendly meal.

◎ You hold on to your muscle well and rarely suffer cravings.

◎ You want to practice being more mindful about food and escape the modern-day psychological construct of meal structure and timing.

If you meet most of these criteria, here is how you should ease into fasting.

Step 1: Start with frequent eating, but begin a nighttime fasting regimen where food is consumed only within a 12-hour time period; we advocate 8:00 a.m. to 8:00 p.m. (You got used to this in the 3-2-1 ELEL approach.)

Step 2: Continue with the 12-hour fast, but reduce your eating frequency to three meals (breakfast, lunch, and dinner) and one preemptive snack. For instance, if you tend to be hungry and have cravings in the evening, eat a small protein and/or nonstarchy vegetable snack at 2:30 or 3:00 p.m.

Step 3: Reduce your meal intake to two or three meals per day. This is almost exactly the 3-2-1 protocol you started with, remember?

Benefit and Downfall

One of the major hidden benefits of fasting is also its major downfall: You will feel hunger as you are exposed to the constant food cues. For almost all beginners, this is too powerful an urge to overcome. This is why we feel fasting is rarely a smart starting place for beginners in the fat-loss lifestyle. But feeling hunger and being mindful of not giving in to urges is something those of us who have fasted previously can do. This is a very beneficial skill to have, but not everyone can do it, and it takes practice.

A Quick Fix

Consider *modified metabolic fasting*. This is a fasting strategy in which certain foods, such as nonstarchy water-based veggies like celery, cucumbers, peppers, and lettuce (which can be eaten whenever) and branched-chain amino acids are used to blunt some of the negative hormonal effects of fasting. Since in our experience women fare worse than men with fasting, these modified fasts are often what we use for female fasters.

Stage 4: If your metabolism is very balanced, or fasting simply appeals to you, eat just one big meal at the end of the day; fast one to three times per week or every other day (alternate-day fasting).

Find the eating pattern that works best for you. The right one should keep you full and satiated, eliminate cravings, and balance your energy. Even with fasting, you always want your HEC in check.

Signs Fasting Is Not Working for You

◎ You feel uncontrollable hunger, energy lows, and strong cravings.

◎ You start noticing that you have difficulty sleeping and/or a feeling that you're "wired but tired" during the day.

◎ You have a "flabby and crabby" metabolism. This is when you become moody and irritable, and you also lose muscle mass and are not as tight as you were before. Your fat distribution also shifts toward your belly.

◎ Your strength and endurance begin to falter. If you are an exerciser and you start noticing your performance decreasing in the gym, this is a sure sign you are not recovering adequately between workouts, and fasting might be working against you. If you are purely seeking fat loss, you may not be too worried about this, but it is an early sign that things may be going south.

◎ A few other self-evaluations you can give yourself are the pupil dilation test, the waking heart rate test, the heart rate recovery test, and, best of all, the heart rate variability test. All of these can give a glimpse into how your nervous system is holding up under the stress of any diet or exercise program, including fasting.

- **Pupil dilation.** Go into a darkened but not completely dark room (you'll need to be able to see your pupils). Shine a small flashlight to the side of your eye and watch your pupils. They should constrict tightly and remain that way for at least 30 to 60 seconds. If they pulsate or dilate again before this, it may indicate adrenal stress. Do this test frequently and compare your results—if you see a drop in the time your pupils are dilated, you might have adrenal stress. You can see this change, and thus the effect fasting may be having. This is a very crude clinical tool we use to assess adrenal stress and is best when done repeatedly so you know your normal non-stressed response. If the test indicates adrenal stress, you should not fast.

- **Waking heart rate.** Take your heart rate first thing in the morning before getting out of bed. An increased rate may indicate overtraining.

- **Heart rate recovery.** HRR is a measure of how fast the heart recovers from exertion and is an indication of nervous system stress. While training, monitor the resiliency of your heart rate recovery. A workout that is too stressful or poor nutrition will result in a less efficient HRR and is an indication that fasting (or any other stressful dietary regimen, with all else being equal) may need to be reconsidered. A normal heart rate recovery is a drop of 20 beats in 60 seconds. Poor diet or overtraining can quickly alter this optimal response. To use this tool, continuously assess your heart rate throughout your workout. This is more easily done when wearing a heart rate monitor. You may find that as a workout progresses, your HRR is diminished. It may be a good idea to end the workout as soon as this happens and reevaluate your eating or lifestyle approach.

- **Heart rate variability.** HRV is one of the newer and more sensitive tools available to health enthusiasts. It measures the time delay between beats of the heart. You may think your heartbeat is predictable and steady like a metronome, but it is actually irregular and varied. In fact, the more varied it is, the healthier you are. It is now possible to find tools that measure this sensitive indicator of sympathetic and parasympathetic balance. Many of these tools can be integrated with a mobile device and give you a wonderful way to assess how stress affects your physiology. Negative effects of stress, exercise, or an eating regimen will show in negative changes in HRV. (Our favorite HRV tool, BioForce HRV, can be found at bioforcehrv.com.)

THE SCIENCE: *Hormones, Fasting, and the Stress Response*

Fasting proponents say skipping meals has no effect on cortisol. Advocates for eating more frequently say skipping meals raises cortisol. The truth is that neither group is totally right. If fasting causes excess stress, one change you will see is a "reverse cortisol curve," in which the normal pattern of starting high in the morning and dropping low in the evening changes to having a cortisol level lower than normal in the morning and higher than normal in the evening. In conversations about stress hormones, cortisol sometimes is used as a catchall for stress reactions. Yes, your cortisol level is raised during stress, but it is often delayed compared to the immediate release of catecholamines (adrenaline and noradrenaline). Cortisol is also often blamed for the long-term consequences of stress regarding weight gain, even though neuropeptide Y (NPY) probably should take some of the blame.

Stress reactions involve more than just cortisol, and any negative stress reactions as a consequence of fasting involve other hormones as well. In many (but again, not

all) people, going without food is a stressor. In response to that stress, the body will release adrenaline and then cortisol. The purpose of this is to raise blood sugar and burn fat. (This is the same thing that happens in short, intense exercise workouts, by the way.) It is wrong to assume that this stress reaction is always a bad thing. In fact, it is this very response that ramps up fat burning and delivers the sometimes hugely beneficial fat loss that some intermittent fasters achieve. However, it is also wrong to assume that this reaction is always a good thing. An overexaggerated adrenaline and cortisol response can lead to muscle wasting in some, as well as hunger, energy fluctuation, and severe cravings that will derail any diet.

This same response, when repeated chronically, causes the sympathetic nervous system to release NPY and elevate the level of ghrelin. These two hormones are what we call the "yo-yo hormones" because they are likely part of the reason why many dieters, including those on fasting programs, end up gaining back more fat than they started with.

And that is the issue with fasting. For some, the total hormonal environment is such that fat is burned and muscle is maintained. For others, fat and muscle might both be lost. For still others, fat may be slow to go and muscle much faster. This is why one person can fast and look great and another can fast and end up flabby, and someone else can fast and lose fat and muscle but have their fat shift to their midsection.

Fasting advocates often point out that ghrelin and human growth hormone (HGH) levels rise with fasting. This is considered positive, but too much ghrelin or HGH is not a good thing. Excess HGH can actually lead to insulin resistance, and too much ghrelin can lead to constant cravings and increased fat-storing potential. Both are a recipe for yo-yo weight regain. What looks like a great solution in the short term can quickly turn into a long-term disaster for fat loss. The major takeaway we want to leave you with is that when it comes to fasting and eating frequency, you should proceed with caution and do what works for you.

THE LOSE WEIGHT HERE RECAP

◎ Vegetables and lean proteins are your best fat-loss foods. You can eat them in almost unlimited quantities.

◎ Wet starches and fattier foods can help you feel satiated when protein and vegetables are not enough. Find your tolerance for each separately.

◎ Don't skip carbs—just understand the different types and how they impact your ability to lose weight. Know when to eat them, which ones to eat, and how much of them to eat. Learn your carb tipping point.

◎ Fasting isn't good for everybody, and the effects can be negative for some. But if you feel you are ready and capable, consider trying it. Done properly—by easing into it and by being aware of how your body reacts—it can be a great fat-loss tool and one of the healthier lifestyle choices.

CHAPTER 9

PRO-SHAPE:

Target the Area

N ow that you have increased fat burning globally by taking care to control the Laws of Metabolic Compensation and Metabolic Multitasking, it is time to teach you some advanced tricks for dealing with stubborn fat. The 3-2-1 and 4-2-2 protocols helped you break the diet cycle and take the brakes off stubborn fat, allowing it to be burned at the same rate as fat in the rest of the body so you can reshape yourself into the coveted hourglass or V shape. But sometimes, even when fat loss from stubborn areas speeds up, it still lags behind the rest of the body. This chapter helps you troubleshoot this issue.

For the sake of simplicity, we will divide stubborn fat into a few specific areas.

1. Female lower-body fat and cellulite

2. Female belly fat

3. Back-of-the-arm fat

4. Male belly fat

5. Love handles

6. Male chest fat

FEMALE LOWER-BODY FAT AND CELLULITE

We'll start with lower-body fat and cellulite. Women tend to carry body fat in the lower body, mainly because of the influence of estrogen, which increases alpha-adrenergic-receptor density in the butt, hip, and thigh regions. In addition, the vertical positioning of female collagen fibers results in fat-cell accumulation inside collagen pockets. This causes the characteristic dimpling and puckering of cellulite. Together these physiological characteristics can result in slow fat release from the lower body and/or issues with cellulite in both overweight and thin women.

Remember, catecholamines are the major drivers of fat loss during exercise. There are two types of receptors catecholamines bind to: alpha-adrenergic receptors and beta-adrenergic receptors. Think of the beta-receptors as fat burners (B for *burn*) and the alpha-receptors as fat storers (A for *anti-burn*). Because women have a much higher percentage of alpha-receptors in their lower bodies, they do not burn fat in this area efficiently. In order to attack this, we want to:

1. Decrease alpha-receptor activity

2. Ramp up beta-receptor stimulation

There are a few ways to block the action of alpha-receptors. First, stop dieting. Hopefully, we have drilled this into you by now. Next, decrease your body's insulin exposure. This reduces alpha-adrenergic-receptor function—that's where the 3-2-1 and 4-2-2 protocols come into play.

In addition, there are some supplement and exercise strategies that can help. Three supplements in particular can make a difference.

1. Green tea extract (GTE)

2. *Coleus forskohlii* (forskolin)

3. Yohimbine HCl

If you recall, catecholamines (adrenaline and noradrenaline, also called epinephrine and norepinephrine) bind to both alpha- and beta-receptors. When they bind to alphas, fat release is slowed or blocked; when they bind to betas, fat release is increased. So any area that has more alphas than betas, like the female lower body, will be resistant as heck to fat loss. But what if you could produce inside a fat cell the same effects that occur when beta-receptors are activated? That is what green tea extract and *Coleus forskohlii* do. They activate the same cellular mechanism involving a compound called cyclic AMP that occurs with beta-receptor activation. In other words, they bypass this receptor issue altogether. But before you start jumping up and down and think you can eat what you want and simply take these supplements, you need to understand that the effect of these supplements is minor and only works when insulin levels are kept in control. You must adhere to the 3-2-1 and 4-2-2 protocols first, and then these supplements can give you a boost. We have used this combination in our clinic so often that we know it works. We also know it works only in conjunction with tight dietary adherence.

There are a few other compounds that seem to be able to directly block alpha-receptor activity. These include yohimbine HCl, synephrine, and berberine. In our clinical experience, yohimbine works best. But there are several caveats to this. Unlike GTE and forskolin, which can be taken daily, yohimbine works only in certain situations: on an empty stomach, before exercise, and when not used continuously. Yohimbine is a stimulant, and the body will adapt to it. Its impact, like that of other supplements, is almost completely negated by the influence of more powerful fat-cell regulators such as insulin. This is why it should be used on an empty stomach. It is also short acting, so you want to take it right before exercise; that way, when the fat-burning catecholamines are released, yohimbine is there to make sure far fewer alpha-receptors are active. We do want to sound a very big caution here: Please *do not* take yohimbine, or any supplement for that matter, without talking to your physician first.

Another great strategy to make sure you burn more fat after an exercise session with yohimbine is to follow the workout with some aerobic exercises. Low-intensity walking for as long as is feasible (preferably 60 to 90 minutes per day) is best because it also lowers cortisol.

As for the dimply appearance of your thighs, there is little you can do to impact the collagen aspect of the problem. Newer medical spa treatments that involve various forms of mechanical massage, laser light, heat, suction, and pressure may have benefits. Foam rolling and hydrotherapy, forms of self-guided deep-tissue massage and blood-flow stimulation, may also be beneficial.

Clinically, some women swear by these methods to eliminate cellulite. We're not sure there is enough evidence to say either way. Plus, the fact that there is little research suggesting they work makes this an unknown. One thing to note: Pretty

The Science of Cellulite

Unlike in men, the collagen fibers in women's lower bodies run vertically, like a picket fence. This straight up-and-down distribution is the major reason females get cellulite and men don't; estimates suggest that 90 percent of women have some degree of cellulite, compared to 10 percent of men. Collagen in men forms more of a mesh—if women have a picket fence distribution, men have the chain link fence distribution. This is an important distinction: Vertical distribution of female collagen fibers forms the pockets in which fat cells grow. As the cells grow in size, they are essentially corralled and packed together tightly by the collagen fibers. This tight packing of fat inside the collagen pockets is what creates cellulite's puckering and dimpling.

Blasting Cellulite

Why do some women have cellulite and others don't? And why do some overweight women have less cellulite than some skinny women? These are great questions, and they underscore the need to move beyond the simple fat-loss models many experts cling to. Cellulite is not just an issue of gaining or losing fat. It is an issue of doing something to address both fat accumulation and collagen strength and health. The reason some women get cellulite and some women don't is mostly due to genetics. Some women have collagen fibers that are more like a man's, and some have extreme versions of the vertical distribution. So getting rid of cellulite is perfectly possible for some women and far more difficult for others.

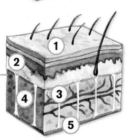

Male Skin

1. Epidermis
2. Dermis
3. Collagen Fibers
4. Fat Cells
5. Muscle

Female Skin

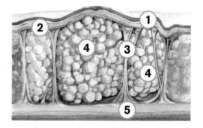

much any massage type of treatment will reduce the appearance of cellulite for a short time given the ability of massage to move lymph and increase blood flow. We think these methods just temporarily shift fluid out of the subcutaneous tissue. (It is believed that fluid, like fat, accumulates in the collagen pockets and can increase the dimpling effect, so removing this fluid may decrease the appearance of dimpling and puckering.) Knowing this is comforting to women who want a quick solution to decreasing the appearance of their cellulite. However, it is a very short-lived effect.

Lower-Body Blast Protocol

Focusing on diet, exercise, and stress reduction is still your best approach to reshaping your lower body.

Diet: Consider sticking to the ELEL approach in lower-estrogen states, which occur in the late luteal phase and early follicular phase of the menstrual cycle (i.e., the week before and the week of your period). Make sure you do more relaxing activities during this time. Do EMEM the other 2 weeks.

Exercise: Do intense 20-minute rest-based intervals or the metabolic chain workouts for 20 minutes followed by low-intensity walking for as long as possible, three to five times a week on an empty stomach. This is what some refer to as *glycogen-depleting exercise.*

Supplements:

- *Coleus forskohlii* (forskolin): 250 milligrams daily (standardized to 20 percent forskolin)

- Green tea extract: 300 milligrams daily (standardized to 45 percent or more EGCG)

Consider a Fat Burner Complex

We sell a product that combines green tea and *Coleus forskohlii* in adequate and standardized doses. While this book is not about trying to sell you supplements, you may want to compare any product you purchase to the one we use clinically with great success. Our supplement is called Fat Burner Complex and can be found online at the Metabolic Effect store (metaboliceffect.com).

- Yohimbine HCl (better than yohimbe bark): 5 to 10 milligrams before fasted exercise; ramp up slowly and make sure you talk to your doctor first.

- Coffee: A cup may give a little extra catecholamine kick during a time when alpha-receptors are blocked, but could be overly stimulating for some when taken with yohimbine.

Cycle It: Remember cycling between the 3-2-1 and 4-2-2 plans? This protocol should be done in cycles of 7 to 14 days on the protocol and 7 to 14 days or longer off the protocol. The EGCG and forskolin can be used daily whether you are on or off the protocol, but the combination of other supplements, like yohimbine, should be used only for short periods of time while on the protocol.

Low-Insulin State versus Glycogen Depletion

We use the terms *low-insulin state* and *glycogen depletion,* which we know may be confusing. The best way to think about a low-insulin state is as a time when you have been without food for 4 to 6 hours or have been eating only veggies and lean protein. The lowest-insulin states occur first thing in the morning, 4 to 6 hours after eating, and at the end of the day on the 3-2-1 protocol, when you have eaten nothing but mostly protein and veggies the whole day.

Glycogen, the stored form of sugar, is stored in your liver and muscles. The purpose of liver glycogen is to supply the brain and body with an easy sugar source when you go without eating. The glycogen in muscle cells can be used only by that muscle for energy when resources are low. If your glycogen stores are constantly filled up, as they are in an Eat More, Exercise Less situation, the body rarely has need to burn fat. This is why many Americans who constantly eat large amounts of starch and sugar, even during an hourlong exercise session (think gel packs and Gatorade), will never lose fat.

Glycogen depletion is a state in which the supply of stored liver and muscle glycogen is lowered to such a degree that the body becomes more reliant on stored fat. Be careful, though: Extreme glycogen depletion caused by cutting out all carbs and exercising like a fiend can cause the body to also lose muscle or to experience metabolic compensation. This is why eating adequate protein, finding your carb tipping point, and training with weights are so critical to your fat-loss efforts.

Supplement Safety

With all of the supplements we're suggesting in this chapter come a few warnings. Some require you to check with your doctor before taking them. Yohimbine, for example, can act as a stimulant and as a monoamine oxidase inhibitor (MAOI), raising the levels of serotonin, adrenaline, and dopamine. Also note that the combination of caffeine and yohimbine can be overly stimulating for some sensitive individuals. Mix and match the supplements according to your sensitivity and start with lower doses. All may not be required, and while the protocol may be less effective without them, it will still be useful.

 ADVANCED CONSIDERATIONS FOR FEMALE LOWER-BODY FAT

As you have learned, estrogen increases alpha-adrenergic-receptor activity. This means that when your estrogen level is higher, such as late in the follicular phase and early in the luteal phase, your lower-body fat is more stubborn. You can use this knowledge to help attack this fat more specifically, and we have a simple method to do so: Attack the lower-body fat more during the luteal phase. Do this by adjusting your supplement intake for the lower-body-fat protocol to coincide with this time.

Conversely, your lowest estrogen levels occur the week before and the week of your period. Make this the time to use the lower-body-fat supplements. Note: Always talk to a physician before making any changes to diet, exercise, and especially supplements.

The current state of research in this area is highly controversial and contradictory. This is largely due to the inability to isolate these effects under the influence of other, more powerful hormonal influences. Hormones do not work in isolation, and estrogen and progesterone are weaker by comparison in their ability to influence fat metabolism. Their influence becomes apparent only when other hormones are controlled. In addition, each woman is different, making research extrapolations more difficult.

FEMALE BELLY FAT

Female belly fat is rarer than male belly fat. This is largely a result of the natural impact of estrogen and progesterone to protect against fat gain in the midsection. Subcutaneous belly fat (just under the skin) and visceral belly fat (deep belly fat) have slightly different properties. Young women typically complain of stubborn subcutaneous belly fat, while older women complain of both visceral and subcutaneous fat.

When we refer to belly fat, we are referring to what is commonly known as an apple-shaped body type, not a pear-shaped one.

Hormonal Impact

Insulin and cortisol exert a strong influence on belly fat in both men and women, with cortisol being more influential in women. Often women with belly fat (meaning increased waist-to-hip ratio) are more stress sensitive and less stress adaptive, especially thin women with belly fat. This can be hard to visualize, so here is a diagram from a study on female belly fat.

This drives home the point that belly fat is not a simple matter of gaining or losing fat. Calories matter, but hormones may matter more when it comes to where we store fat and how to attack our uniquely stubborn areas of body fat. If you are a woman doing everything right and you still struggle with belly fat—especially if you're thin—you need to understand that the primary issue for you is stress management. It's not too many calories. It's not too many carbs. It's not because you are not doing enough exercise. It is stress.

Source: Epel, McEwen, Seeman, Matthews, Castellazzo, et al. "Stress and Body Shape: Stress-Induced Cortisol Secretion Is Consistently Greater Among Women with Central Fat." *Psychosomatic Medicine* 62 (2000): 623–32.

Estrogen and progesterone together block the negative influences of insulin and cortisol on belly fat. They are the reasons women tend to have a lower incidence of belly fat than men. But in women who do have belly fat, it is normally caused by lower-than-normal estrogen and progesterone levels. The most common reasons for these hormonal changes: chronic stress and menopause. Both stress and menopause create a hormonal imbalance that is lower in estrogen, higher in testosterone, and higher in cortisol and insulin. Another common condition that paints a very similar hormonal picture is polycystic ovarian syndrome (PCOS). Compared with other lean women, lean women with PCOS have significantly more fat storage in the belly. So women with PCOS should pay very close attention to our belly fat discussion.

To combat belly fat, we have two main strategies:

1. Relax the body and decrease stress hormones, especially cortisol.

2. Make the body as insulin sensitive as possible by using smart nutrition and exercise.

What Is Stress?

Stress is not just unpleasant, high-pressure, at-the-office anxiety. It is all of that, but it is also experienced by a new mother at home with a little baby, sleep deprived and nutritionally depleted. She is probably more stressed out than anyone else despite the fact that she's probably thrilled and happy.

Combating Stress

Since belly fat can mostly be attributed to stress, consider any and all rest and recovery activities that lower stress:

◎ Make sleep a priority.

◎ Get 1 extra hour of sleep.

◎ Get a massage.

◎ Take a luxurious bath.

◎ Take a nap.

◎ Have sex.

Belly Blast Protocol

Exercise, diet, and supplements together can help target belly fat. We suggest:

Diet and Exercise: The 3-2-1 protocol is best for a belly-fat blast.

Supplements:

- A daily metabolic multivitamin that includes high-dose B vitamins and chromium. This will help combat insulin resistance and replace resources that stress depletes, especially zinc, magnesium, and vitamin B_6.

- Green coffee extract: 1,000 milligrams daily. Like green tea extract, this is an insulin-sensitizing supplement.

- Berberine: Two to four 500 milligram doses daily. Berberine may work against alpha-adrenergic receptors and outperformed metformin for insulin issues associated with PCOS in one study. We have seen great success with this compound clinically.

- Curcumin (we suggest the Meriva formulation): 1,000 to 4,000 milligrams daily. This helps the metabolic command and control center, the hypothalamus and pituitary glands, react better to stress. It also blocks major enzymes involved in fat storage (fatty acid synthase) and the resistance to losing belly fat (11ß-hydroxysteroid dehydrogenase) and may have a positive impact on ovarian function in women with PCOS.

BACK-OF-THE-ARM FAT

One other area of troublesome fat for females is the backs of the arms. We warn you that this may be the most difficult fat of all to deal with. The problem—what makes it so pesky and challenging—is that we don't actually know what causes it. Unlike female lower-body fat and belly fat, arm fat has not been very well researched. What we do know: Subcutaneous fat is much richer in alpha-receptors than beta-receptors. We also know female subcutaneous fat is richer in alpha-receptors than male subcutaneous fat. What we don't know is why some women have troublesome arm fat and so many others do not.

We have deduced some tips for combating arm fat in our clinical practice, but this is no substitute for good research. While we have had some success with arm fat, it has been far less pronounced than our success in getting rid of lower-body fat and belly fat.

One of the things we have noticed is that our patients with PCOS tend to be very heavy in the middle of the body, with pronounced abdominal areas and less fat in the lower body. A 2008 study published in *Gynecological Endocrinology* confirmed our findings. We have also noticed that these women tend to have tighter and leaner triceps. We have always assumed that leaner arms and legs with a greater amount of belly fat is caused by higher testosterone levels. At the same time, we noticed our patients with hypothyroidism have the exact opposite issue: They tend to have higher amounts of neck and arm fat.

We have found that these women can lessen flabbiness in these areas with weight training. So our protocol for female arm fat is one that tries to address the potential hypothyroid issue while raising testosterone naturally with weight training. It also uses the same supplement approach as the female lower-body-fat protocol.

Diet: Follow the 3-2-1 protocol.

Exercise: Follow the 3-2-1 protocol, but add one more exercise specific to toning and tightening the triceps muscles, such as a close-grip pushup. Complete 2 to 5 minutes of close-grip pushups either before or after you complete the regular workout. This exercise does nothing to burn fat, but it can can tighten and shape the triceps, making the area less jiggly. Fair warning: A 2- to 5-minute set of close-grip pushups will challenge the fittest person on the planet. So go slow and use the rest-based training method. If done correctly, toward the end you will be able to do only 1 rep at a time. Here's how: Get in a normal pushup position but place your hands side by side directly under your chest, rather than under your shoulders. Start on your toes, but shift onto your knees if that gets too difficult. You can also stand facing a wall and push off from it using the same technique if you need an easier version.

Note: Consider having your thyroid levels checked or your medication adjusted with your physician.

Supplements: This regimen will be pretty much the same as the supplement suggestions for lower-body fat (see page 197 for dosages):

1. Green tea extract

2. *Coleus forskohlii* (forskolin)

3. Yohimbine HCl

TARGETING ACCORDING TO A WOMAN'S CYCLE

There are two distinct phases of the menstrual cycle. The follicular phase is marked by the beginning of menses (day 1 of the cycle) and ends at ovulation (approximately day 14). It is called the follicular phase because a follicle containing an egg is maturing at that time, mainly under the influence of follicle-stimulating hormone. The proper maturation of this follicle is essential for the release of an egg.

The second phase of the cycle is the luteal phase. This phase is marked by ovulation and the subsequent transformation of the follicle into the corpus luteum once the egg is released. This phase is triggered by a large surge in luteinizing hormone, which causes the follicle to "pop" and release its egg. The corpus luteum becomes the major source of progesterone. If the egg is not fertilized, the corpus luteum degrades, estrogen and progesterone levels fall, and the uterine lining is shed.

What Does This Have to Do with Fat Loss?

As we've mentioned before, in addition to having reproductive functions, estrogen and progesterone impact fat storage and fat burning. This is mainly because they can mildly influence two primary fat-regulating hormones: insulin and cortisol.

Estrogen decreases insulin's impact on the fat-storing enzyme lipoprotein lipase, making the body more sensitive to insulin. The overall impact of estrogen is less fat storage and enhanced fat burning. Estrogen is also anti-cortisol (as is progesterone). Therefore, the follicular phase of the menstrual cycle, when estrogen is higher, allows a greater tolerance for insulin-promoting foods (i.e., starchy foods). It also makes the body more resistant to stressful forms of exercise that cause muscle loss, like long-duration cardio.

The follicular phase of the menstrual cycle is a great time to focus on steady-state, longer-duration, moderate-intensity cardiovascular exercise and more intense weight training. In other words, it's the best time to engage in an Eat More, Exercise More (EMEM) approach. This combination will enhance fat loss and maintain or perhaps even trigger lean muscle gains due to estrogen's effects during this time. Some research also hints that the early follicular phase may produce the best performance outcomes for athletic women.

Progesterone works against the action of estrogen and may make the body more insulin resistant, resulting in your having a greater chance of storing fat and losing muscle. Based on these metabolic considerations, women should watch their starch and sugar intake during the luteal phase and minimize more stressful forms of exercise. With progesterone relatively higher than estrogen in the luteal phase, the female metabolism is more reliant on sugar compared to fat metabolism.

These luteal phase changes create a great opportunity to use the 3-2-1 approach, pairing traditional weight training with lots of leisure activities. By focusing on weight training and lots of walking, we can overcome the slowdown in fat loss by "starving the fat" with much lower calorie intake, but maintain muscle with elevated protein intake and heavy weight lifting.

One caveat regarding this approach is that, due to the primacy of insulin and cortisol, a woman with high insulin and/or cortisol levels (such as those who eat a standard American high-starch diet) who is insulin resistant will not see the pronounced effect of this style of training, because insulin and cortisol are far

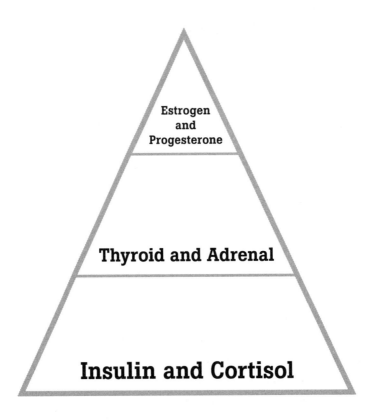

```
        Estrogen
          and
      Progesterone

    Thyroid and Adrenal

    Insulin and Cortisol
```

stronger promoters of fat than either estrogen or progesterone. We use a pyramid diagram to illustrate this concept.

This protocol works with women undergoing normal menstrual cycles who are not using hormonal birth control methods and are living relatively low-insulin-promoting lifestyles or using the 3-2-1 or 4-2-2 approach. Because insulin and cortisol are stronger and at the base of the "metabolic totem pole" compared to estrogen and progesterone, their influence could essentially negate any beneficial influence exerted by the reproductive hormones. The same is true for hormonal oral contraceptive pills (OCP) and hormone replacement therapy (HRT). Giving static doses of hormones completely eliminates the natural cycling nature that this protocol takes advantage of, as OCP and HRT mimic the luteal phase of the menstrual cycle.

Exercise and Diet:

    1. Follicular phase (days 1 to 14): Use the 4-2-2 approach. Do metabolic chain workouts four times weekly and rest-based intervals along with walking or a couple of traditional cardio sessions twice weekly.

2. **Luteal phase (day 15 to menses):** Use the 3-2-1 approach. Do four sets with 10 repetitions of full-body traditional weight training (squat, bench press, back row, shoulder press), two times weekly, and leisure walking on all or most days of the week.

MALE BELLY FAT

Whereas female belly fat does best with the more restorative 3-2-1 protocol, male belly fat responds more favorably to the 4-2-2 protocol.

Want to know the formula for a six-pack? It's $(P + V) \times (Sl + IE)$. Protein (P) and vegetables (V) add a high-powered hunger-suppressing punch with little insulin production. This means you consume fewer calories and achieve better hormone balance. Sleep (Sl) magnifies this effect by lowering cortisol and increasing human growth hormone (HGH), a fat-burning and muscle-building hormone. Throw in intense exercise (IE) that favors weight training and interval training (which produce more HGH and testosterone) over long-duration cardio (which produces more cortisol) and you have the recipe for a six-pack.

Your fix lies in replacing sugar and starch with fiber and raising protein consumption while normalizing fat. The foods with the highest ratio of fiber relative to starch are the nonstarchy vegetables; you will want to shoot for nine servings per day. One of the biggest mistakes many make when looking for a tight six-pack is mistaking starches like beans, corn, and potatoes for vegetables. These foods are wet starches, which certainly can work in small amounts, but here they need to take a backseat to nonstarchy vegetables. Review Chapter 8 and become very familiar with the "green" fat-loss foods. You want to focus on these.

One of the main suggestions we give men is that they should increase their protein intake to shut down hunger and cravings. Many men don't eat enough protein, and this is why they frequently find themselves heading to a burger joint to satisfy their hunger and cravings. Foods high in protein include eggs and all lean cuts of meat; cheese and yogurts, while high in protein, can be overdone, which is why they are listed as yellow foods in Chapter 8 and should be regulated to really attack belly fat.

Exercise: A 4-2-2 Approach

Monday, Tuesday, Thursday, and Friday

◎ Do 20 minutes of metabolic chain workouts (see pages 122 to 127).

◎ Don't take structured rests; instead, push until you can't and rest until you can.

◎ See how many rounds you can finish in 20 minutes.

Wednesday and Saturday

◎ Do 20 minutes of rest-based interval training.

◎ Do a 20-second full-exertion sprint followed by slow-motion rest for as long as is required.

◎ Do a 30-second full-exertion sprint followed by slow-motion rest for as long as is required.

◎ Do a 40-second full-exertion sprint followed by slow-motion rest for as long as is required.

◎ Do a 60-second full-exertion sprint followed by slow-motion rest for as long as is required.

◎ Repeat this sequence for 20 minutes, completing as many rounds as possible.

Sunday

◎ Rest.

Daily

◎ Don't forget to walk daily—20,000 steps if possible—and get more than 8 hours of sleep per night.

 ## LOVE HANDLES

Men and, to a lesser extent, women often find that fat stores on the sides of the midsection and lower back—the so-called love handles—are especially resistant to fat loss.

This phenomenon may be a result of the unique physiology of the fat stored in this area. This subcutaneous abdominal fat has special properties that include decreased adipose tissue blood flow, increased insulin sensitivity (which triggers more fat storage and less fat release), and decreased catecholamine sensitivity (decreased fat burning).

Hormones and Love Handles

As it does in all stubborn fat areas, insulin causes increased fat storage and decreased fat release from fat cells because it stimulates the major fat-storing enzyme lipoprotein lipase and inhibits the major fat-releasing enzyme hormone-sensitive lipase. This subcutaneous fat is thus more insulin reactive and accumulates more easily, which makes it harder to burn off.

To combat love handles, we have three goals:

1. Decrease insulin.

2. Block the alpha-adrenergic receptors.

3. Ramp up beta-adrenergic-receptor stimulation.

To do this, we have constructed the following plan:

Diet: A low-starch diet of less than 125 grams per day of carbohydrates from all sources. This may confuse you a bit since we have rarely given specific amounts to shoot for in this book. Don't worry: We still want you to use the structured flexibility concept. If this amount of carbs is too low (you'll know if your HEC goes out of whack), then adjust it. You can think of a cup of rice or a potato as about 30 grams of carbs, so if you stick to the 4-2-2 protocol, you will be hitting this amount almost perfectly without even trying. However, given that love handles are some of the most stubborn fat stores on the body, you may want to eventually get very specific about carb intake and adjust the timing of your carbs as well.

Supplements:

◉ *Coleus forskohlii* (forskolin): 250 milligrams daily (standardized to 20 percent forskolin)

◉ Green tea extract: 300 milligrams daily (standardized to 45 percent or more EGCG)

◉ Yohimbine HCl (better than yohimbe bark): 5 to 10 milligrams (on an empty stomach only before exercise)

◎ 1 cup drip coffee or 150 to 200 milligrams caffeine (on an empty stomach before exercise)

Exercise: Start with 20 minutes of rest-based intervals or 20 minutes of metabolic chain workouts followed by low-intensity walking for as long as possible (preferably 60 to 90 minutes). Do this three to five times per week, preferably on an empty stomach.

Cycle It: Remember cycling between the 3-2-1 and 4-2-2 plans? This protocol should be done in cycles lasting 7 to 14 days on the protocol and 7 to 14 days or longer off the protocol. The EGCG and forskolin can be used daily whether you are on or off the protocol, but the combination of other supplements, like yohimbine, should be used only for short periods of time while on the protocol.

MALE CHEST FAT

Often referred to as "man boobs," chest fat may be the most distressing fat men deal with. The good news is that it is not nearly as stubborn as love handles and usually can be dealt with simply by following the 3-2-1 or 4-2-2 protocol outlined in this book.

When that is not the case, however, you will need to focus on two hormones: testosterone and estrogen. This protocol attempts to raise the former while lowering the latter.

There are several things that we can tell you have worked very well clinically. You may be surprised to know that popular herbs and supplements on the market that claim to raise testosterone levels are not among them. If you have been interested in raising your testosterone level naturally, you have likely heard of *Tribulus terrestris,* deer antler velvet, and other testosterone "boosters." We have looked at enough before-and-after lab values of male patients using these compounds to say with confidence that they are useless in raising testosterone. (Happily, research supports our clinical experience.)

However, there are two supplements we do notice an impact with. Minerals such as zinc and magnesium and vitamin D can make a difference, especially if you are deficient—and we find that upward of 70 percent of men in our clinical practice are indeed deficient in one or more of these nutrients. If you are among that 70 percent, supplementing will likely have an impact. This is what we have seen clinically, and the research also validates us on this point.

The other supplement is an aromatase inhibitor. Aromatase is an enzyme in the body that converts testosterone into estrogen. In many men with lower testosterone levels, this enzyme has a high rate of activity. There are reliable natural aromatase inhibitors that we use in our clinic daily; some of the better ones include chrysin, nettle, pygeum, and saw palmetto. Many of these same compounds block another testosterone-impacting enzyme called 5-alpha reductase. If you would like to see the compound we use in our clinical practice, check out the formula for our product called Androgen Complex at metaboliceffect .com/product/androgen-complex.

Diet: Follow the 3-2-1 and 4-2-2 cycling protocol.

Exercise: Follow the 3-2-1 and 4-2-2 cycling protocol.

Supplements:

◎ Vitamin D:
  - If your blood level is above 50 nanograms per milliliter, take 2,000 IU daily in winter.
  - If your blood level is below 50 nanograms per milliliter, take 2,000 to 5,000 IU daily until your level rises above 50 nanograms per milliliter.
  - If your blood level is below 30 nanograms per milliliter, talk to your doctor about taking 10,000 IU or more daily until your level rises.

◎ Zinc: Take 20 to 30 milligrams daily (the best formulations are zinc aspartate and zinc citrate).

◎ Magnesium: Take 300 to 600 milligrams daily of an easily absorbed form, such as magnesium glycinate or magnesium aspartate.

◎ Saw palmetto: Take 400 milligrams (standardized to contain 45 percent fatty acids).

◎ Pygeum: Take 200 milligrams daily (standardized to contain 12 percent phytosterols).

◎ Nettle: Take 200 milligrams daily (standardized to contain 0.8 percent beta-sitosterol).

◎ Chrysin: Take 50 ßeta-sitosterol daily.

THE LOSE WEIGHT HERE RECAP

You can target really stubborn body fat by blasting it with a combination of diet, exercise, and supplements. Primarily the 3-2-1 and 4-2-2 protocols will aid in these areas.

There are some keys to blasting each.

- Female lower-body fat: Do spurts of high-intensity exercise followed by long walks on an empty stomach. Time your diet cycling and supplement intake with lower-estrogen times.

- Cellulite: This comes down mostly to genetics. Be wary of spas that promise to reduce it, though some of their treatments can reduce the dimply appearance for a short time.

- Female belly fat: Work on stress reduction.

- Back-of-the-arm fat: While the cause of this remains a mystery, consider adding 2 to 5 minutes of close-grip pushups to your workouts to firm and tighten this area.

- Target to your menstrual cycle: Switch to a 3-2-1 protocol during the 2 weeks following ovulation, and use the 4-2-2 protocol during the 2 weeks after the start of a period. But if you are also trying to target lower-body fat, consider focusing your supplement use during the week before and during your period.

- Male belly fat: Eat a six-pack protein and vegetable diet, and exercise intensely with a mix of weights and intervals.

- Love handles: Cycle your diet and exercise between the 3-2-1 and 4-2-2 protocols, go a little lower-carb with your diet, and use targeted supplements. That is the key to love-handle reshaping.

- Male chest fat: Raise testosterone levels and lower estrogen levels by lowering aromatase and stimulating testosterone production.

Conclusion

I f you made it this far, hopefully you've learned that the only viable option for sustainable weight loss is working with, rather than against, your metabolism. Most important, though, is that you've learned how metabolism really works, and why having this understanding is so critical to burning fat and changing your shape for good.

Remember: There is no diet you can find, there is only the diet you create. You don't follow a plan—you build a lifestyle. That means you will always need to tweak, adjust, and recalibrate your approach as you inch closer to finding the exact formula that works for you. It may be exactly what is outlined in this book, but more likely it will end up deviating from it substantially.

If you are not ready to accept this fact, then you are not really ready to give up the dieter mentality and will soon find yourself reading once again about the next great diet craze and trying to fit yourself into a broken model that fails almost everyone.

Please don't make that mistake.

WILLPOWER IS NOT THE TOOL YOU WANT TO LEAN ON

You might think now all you need to do is muster all your willpower and run off to follow the plan in this book. Let this be the final key insight we want to impress upon you: Willpower is not what you want. What you want is *skillpower*. Understanding the difference is critical.

Research has shown that willpower is like a battery: It can be drained, and it can be recharged. Most people have willpower batteries that are so small and so drained they are ill equipped to make even a single change without failing.

How do you switch from a drained resource called willpower to the fully charged one called skillpower? There are a few key exercises we'll show you now. Once you master these skills, you'll find you have a supercharged, mega-sized battery of skillpower available to you.

The Three Batteries

We like to think of your willpower battery as being made up of three small batteries.

◎ Mental battery

◎ Physical battery

◎ Emotional battery

Each of these batteries has its own reserves, and together they determine the size and charge of your willpower battery. All three must be charged and in balance to make sure your willpower can grow and hold a charge for a long time.

Let's look at a real-life example. Take your stereotypical stressed-out, overworked, sleep-deprived businessperson. At some point he or she made a choice, whether consciously or unconsciously, to keep the mental battery charged at the expense of the physical and emotional batteries. Because of that, this person ended up overweight and unhealthy—and with broken friendships and family relationships to boot.

Can you relate? Let's take a look at your smaller batteries.

The Mental Battery

This battery is easily drained and as a result, when it's depleted, it will drain the willpower battery as well. Since each battery can steal energy from the others, this one will frequently tap the physical and emotional batteries to charge up. Without proper balance and knowledge, this can result in choosing quick energy sources devoid of high-quality nutrients, such as sugar-based foods and stimulants. It can also mean you have less desire to exercise, since movement requires a mental energy investment in the beginning before it gives back and charges you up.

Since stress shuts down the motivation centers and increases the brain's reward-seeking behaviors, the mental battery is the one most heavily taxed by it. Any form of self-editing or planning drains this battery. By *self-editing*, we mean thinking about trying to control your actions or judging yourself. Obviously, humans do this all the time. But it's those who engage in the greatest amount of internal dialogue and may even think they are doing themselves a favor by worrying about their lives who are draining their mental batteries and their willpower the quickest. The same goes for planning and constantly thinking about all the things you must do. Research shows that this kind of thinking increases the drain on mental power and willpower: The more you try to change about yourself and your life at one time, and the more to-dos you have on your list, the less likely you are to do anything at all. *All or nothing* almost always becomes *nothing*.

Easy Meditation Practice

Set a timer for 5 to 10 minutes. Now, with your eyes shut or open—whichever you choose—become an observer of your body. Watch, listen, and feel as sounds, feelings, visions, and experiences come in and out of the present moment. You can do this while you're driving (eyes open, obviously!), in the shower, while you're cooking, when you're at your desk—pretty much anywhere. Watch things arise and watch them go, coming in and out of your conscious awareness. If you get stuck on a thought, idea, vision, or sound, recognize that and let it go. When your timer goes off, you are done. You can then return to self-editing, planning, and judging, although after this mindfulness practice you will find you are less and less likely to do these things.

Mindful meditation is wonderful to use whenever you feel an urge or a trigger tickling you, especially hunger or cravings. One of the best descriptions we have heard for fighting urges is the idea of "surfing the urge." Most people feel that sensations like hunger and cravings are like itches—if they don't scratch them, they will get worse. The truth is they are almost always like waves: They rise, peak in intensity, and then crash and dissipate. The trick is to learn not to get pummeled by the wave, but rather to catch it and surf it without giving in to it, letting it arrive, peak, and go. The more you practice this skill, the greater control you will have over your willpower, and the bigger the charge your willpower battery will hold.

Try these steps to make sure your mental battery is strong.

◎ Focus on changing one aspect of your life at a time.

◎ Write down tasks you need to do rather than holding them in your head. Try to limit this list to the three most important items. Don't attempt to add anything to your to-do list unless you have removed at least two other things first.

◎ Get adequate sleep, move regularly, and engage in plenty of rest and recovery activities. This will reset your mental focus and charge your mental battery.

◎ Practice mindful meditation, one of the best skills to add to your arsenal. So the first item on that list of three important items? *Learn how to meditate.*

The Social MVP Exercise

Think of your friends and family the way you would if you were a professional sports recruiter trying to put together the best team in the history of your league. To do that, you need to make sure your players are in the right positions, and that any empty positions are filled with the best of the best.

Here is how to do it.

Grab a sheet of paper and write down the names of the 10 to 20 people in your social circle who are closest to you.

Draw a table with two columns and three rows, forming six blocks.

◎ In the upper left block, write "Agenda Stealers."

◎ In the upper right block, write "Agenda Saviors."

◎ In the middle left block, write "Emotional Trapdoors."

◎ In the middle right block, write "Emotional Ladders."

◎ In the bottom left block, write "Energy Vampires."

◎ In the bottom right block, write "Energy Spark Plugs."

Agenda Categories. If you had to use your mental battery to focus on a task like solving a problem or meeting a deadline, who on your list would drain you or prevent you from accomplishing it? That's your Agenda Stealer. Who would pitch in and help you directly with the task or take on something else to free you up to accomplish it? That's your Agenda Savior.

Emotional Categories. Who on your list drains your emotional battery after you talk with them? The conversation may contain

The Physical Battery

This entire book has been about the physical battery because it is by far the most important of the three. Illness in the body will sap mental and emotional energy and drain willpower faster than anything else. This is the major reason people desire vitality and health; on some level, they know and understand that when their physical battery is functioning optimally, everything else is substantially easier to manage.

This is why eating in a way that does not deprive or stress out your body is critical. This is why achieving optimal body composition and burning off the fat that weighs you down and eats away at your health and vitality is so important.

---

a lot of "drama," or you may feel weighed down, sad, or tired after talking with them. That's your emotional trapdoor. Who on your list makes you feel encouraged, motivated, or "light" after talking with them? They may even raise your self-esteem. That's your Emotional Ladder.

Energy Categories. Who on your list drains your physical battery? Do you feel physically tired after you've spent time with them? That's your Energy Vampire. Who on your list increases your physical energy? That's your Energy Spark Plug.

Now fill in the blocks with the people on your list. Some people may be in multiple categories and some in none. Who belongs in what category? This is not a character judgment, and no category is necessarily good or bad.

When you're finished, analyze your table and look for patterns.

◎ Is the left column loaded up while the right column is bare?

◎ Do you have too many Agenda Stealers?

◎ Do you have enough people to lift you up and bolster your emotions?

Take some time to notice the people who help or hurt your fat-loss efforts, or any goal, for that matter. When the situation requires, engage with or avoid these people based on your needs and your knowledge of their influence. This can be a critical aspect of reaching your goals. Often it may be helpful to recruit new social team members or avoid others altogether.

It is also why being not just thin but also fit and strong is so critical. With this book, we have given you all the tools necessary to build a big, strong, and robust physical battery that can power your emotional and mental batteries during times of stress and hardship.

Just remember one key warning: Dieting is not a smart move for your physical battery. Remember the metabolic credit card concept? Short-term gain (or in this case, weight loss) leads to long-term penalties and debt. Besides, the miserable self-editing process of dieting also saps the mental battery. That is why we have stressed so strongly in this book that you can't rely on meal plans, recipes, and structured calorie solutions that require you to think about everything you do. Being more intuitive in your approach is better for your willpower battery.

The Emotional Battery

This one might be the hardest to manage because it is strongly influenced by others. Researchers now know that obesity is in a sense contagious—but so is leanness. You tend to be about the same size as the five to ten people you hang around with the most. That is why having a strong emotional support system that not only supports but also engages in your efforts to get and stay healthy with you is critical.

We often fail to realize that it is our responsibility to help ourselves. The idea that everyone around us will always consider our needs is simply not true or realistic. Most of the time these people are consciously or unconsciously seeking our support as well.

We do an exercise with our patients that we find is a very powerful way to strengthen your emotional support system and charge your emotional battery. It has applications for the other batteries as well, as you will see. We call this "The Social MVP Exercise" (pages 216 to 217).

Research has shown that there are other actions that will bolster your emotional battery.

Give more. But be careful—giving with the expectation of getting something in return is a setup for draining your emotional battery. Get in the habit of doing kind, compassionate things without expectation. We love to tip big or just anonymously pay for the coffee of a person in line behind us. But give sporadically instead of all at once: Volunteers who set aside 1 day a week for giving feel more recharged than those who give daily, who end up feeling drained.

Practice gratitude. At the end of every day, list three things for which you are grateful. More importantly, at the end of a day, week, or month when everything seems to be going wrong, think about what you have to be grateful for at that moment. There is always something, and research shows this keeps your emotional battery charged.

Pamper yourself. Often, we make the crucial mistake of attaching our needs to others. Then we are sad, resentful, or angry when the person does not act on it in the way we seek. Whenever you have negative feelings toward a person, or positive feelings of admiration, consider that person a mirror into your own higher self. What you will find is that what you love or hate about them—and the needs you are hoping they will fulfill—are the things you love or hate about or need for yourself. Spend time with yourself to understand what it is you need to be giving, saying, and doing for yourself.

One my favorite things to do (Jade, here) is to take a long weekend away by myself and hang out at a spa, eat at the best restaurants, and treat myself to a mini vacation. There are lots of ways to do this to fit your budget and schedule; find a way that recharges you emotionally and lets you tap in to your higher self.

THREE WILLPOWER PRACTICES

There is one other aspect of willpower we want to teach you about that the entire dieting industry gets wrong. Imagine you are being attacked by a dog that is biting your forearm as you try to shield yourself. (Not a pleasant thought, we know, but stick with us here.) What most people would do is try to pull away from the dog, which will only convince the dog to attack harder and cause more damage.

The better approach would be to shove your forearm toward the dog. This would make it far more likely that the dog would let you go and far less likely that you would be as badly injured as you would have been. We are huge dog lovers, but this illustration serves our point well: What we avoid or pull away from will find us and often do more damage. What we confront head-on becomes known to us, and we quickly learn to beat it.

This is the way you need to start thinking about food. Dieting is not just detrimental to your metabolism; it destroys your psyche too. The ridiculous notion peddled by the health and fitness industry that you just need to suck it up, have more willpower, and never enjoy what you love is exactly the *wrong* approach. It is as detrimental to your psyche as dieting is to your metabolism.

The right approach? Attack the problem head-on. I (Jade, here) absolutely love sweets and pastries and those kinds of things. I know—strange for a "diet guy," right? But I do. They are my weakness. After struggling with this for 20 years, I finally came up with a solution that made me kick the habit within a few months. Instead of forcing myself never to order dessert (which resulted in my feeling deprived, then eating almost an entire cheesecake once a week), I started getting dessert every single time I ate out. However, my new rule was to take only three bites of it.

Guess what happened? I started not liking dessert that much. I also started seeing myself as a person who only ever eats three bites of sweets. Many in the world of psychology call this the as-if principle. As humans, we are sometimes a little less sharp than we think we are. We tend to believe that we decide who we are and then take actions in line with that. Surprisingly, research shows that it works far more strongly in completely the other direction: When we see ourselves taking a particular action, our minds then decide what it means and justify why we are doing it.

So my brain said, "Hmmm, I am eating a dessert, and I am taking only three bites. That must mean I never finish my dessert. I am a person who never finishes dessert. That is who I am." I convinced my brain it was true. You can do that by repeating an action as well.

In her wonderful book *The Willpower Instinct,* Kelly McGonigal, PhD, calls this idea a willpower challenge. It is like giving your willpower muscle a workout, making it stronger and more resilient for its next challenge. In other words, it makes the willpower (or in our case, skillpower) battery larger and increases its charge. We have never seen anything more effective than this to help develop greater skillpower.

Skillpower Workouts

Here are three exercises for building skillpower, from the easiest to the hardest.

Willpower Workout Level 1: The 1-Fry Grab

We learned this from fitness and mind-set expert Jill Coleman (Jade's wife). If someone you often eat with loves to order french fries, allow yourself 1 fry off his or her plate (ask permission first!). This technique also works with 1 bite of dessert or a small bite of chocolate. Many people who have successfully made weight management a lifestyle use this strategy.

Willpower Workout Level 2: The 3-Bite Rule

This is an exercise in which you order something solely for yourself, but limit the amount you eat, like Jade did with desserts. Maybe it's a dessert, a side of onion rings, or potato chips. Whatever it is, don't deprive yourself—just limit your intake.

Willpower Workout Level 3: The Take-Home Challenge

Buy something you love, like a pizza, a huge chocolate bar, or a pint of ice cream, and bring it home with you. Then limit yourself to one serving until the next day. This means that temptation will be sitting there, calling to you, and you must resist its urge. This one is the hardest, and when you master it you have finally become one of those people you envy: a person who seems to have an iron will (or skill).

One tip here: Remember the attacking dog? If you are overwhelmed by the urge to eat more, get out the take-home item. Look at it. Smell it. Feel it, and watch the urge well up in you and start to peak. Then surf it and let it fall and dissipate.

One study on women who were given boxes of chocolates to carry around with them all day showed how powerful this approach is. One group was told they should avoid the chocolates and try to use distraction techniques to keep from eating them, and the other group was told to take the chocolates out, smell and look at them, and engage with them. Guess who ended up eating the most chocolates? The group trying to use the old, worn-out method prescribed by the dieting dictators—sheer willpower. Avoidance and distraction make the urge come back to bite you harder.

FINAL THOUGHTS

The standard dieting model of Eat Less, Exercise More does not work for the vast majority of people because it works against the natural compensatory tendency of metabolism and treats you as if you are the same as every other human on the planet.

The entire purpose of this book was to help you understand that there is no perfect diet out there. The perfect diet is instead a lifestyle that you build using a deep understanding of your own metabolism, psychology, and personal preferences. A lifestyle that you can own, love, and live with—with relative ease.

Your goal now is simple: practice, practice, practice. There is an old saying that practice makes perfect. We, however, prefer "Practice makes progress." The idea of perfection is a myth. In fact, in every other area of life, we understand intuitively that to learn and master something we must fall down, get scraped up, pick ourselves up, dust ourselves off, and learn the lesson to get better.

What we are saying is that you will fail. It is inevitable. Those failures are actually required in order for you to grow, learn, and master the workings of your metabolism. We have this very wrong idea in our culture that success and failure are opposites. They are actually synergistic; that is, you can't have one without the other. We have found that it is those who embrace this concept who make it, and those who don't who ultimately slip back into the mind-set of a dieter and never achieve true change.

So what we would like to leave you with is this: We hope you fail, we hope you fail fast, and we hope you fail a lot, especially in the beginning. That's because we know that if you do, you will get back up each time and use the methods we have taught you to understand your own metabolism, and in the end you will be effortlessly healthy, vibrant, and lean.

What we hope this book has given you, more than anything else, is permission to throw out all the nutrition rules and start over by constructing your own. There is only one rule in nutrition that is true, and that is to do what works for *you*.

As you move forward with this new information, please remember there is still so much we do not understand about nutrition and metabolism, which is why ignorance is acceptable but arrogance is not. Avoid the temptation to pick a nutrition team and instead create your own. Your sanity and health will thank you for it.

The journey does not end, and you will never arrive. You will know you have succeeded when arrival is no longer the goal.

We wish you the very best in health, fitness and vitality,

Jade and Keoni

Mary

Mary accomplished in 10 weeks what she struggled to do in 15 years. A yo-yo dieter, Mary couldn't find anything that worked for her. She had a hard time shaking the weight she gained from two pregnancies. The fat was stubborn and totaled 50 pounds. She had a library full of diet and exercise books and disks, but nothing helped. When she came across the Lose Weight Here program, everything changed. She marveled at the results she saw in just a few weeks and eventually lost 10 inches and 16 pounds.

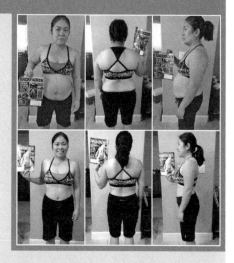

The big change Mary made was with carbs, which used to be the focal point of every meal. She shifted her plate to focus on protein and fiber instead. She also learned to properly fuel her meals pre-workout and replenish postworkout.

Mary says she still has weight to lose, but she's changed her relationship with food and is no longer intimidated by the weight-loss journey. Working out was never Mary's issue. She spent an hour a day in the gym. It was the eating she had really never grasped until she got on this plan, plus she is a foodie who loves trying new restaurants and types of food. She says LWH has been life-changing because not only can she enjoy good food, the plan also fits into her busy life of chasing two toddlers around.

Acknowledgments

We would like to express our deepest thanks and gratitude to our father and mother, Jim and Joyce Teta: for sacrificing so much of yourselves, for teaching, for loving unconditionally, for inspiring us, and for keeping us laughing. Oh, and for giving us names that make everyone think we are husband and wife instead of brothers. They certainly never forget our names. Even though Mom can no longer speak a coherent sentence and Dad frequently gets stuck in place for 2 hours while trying to finish the Sudoku puzzle, we promise we are only a little embarrassed by you. XO

To our wives, Jill Coleman and Jillian Sarno Teta: You are our best friends and we love you both very much. Thank you for your constant counsel and education, and for letting us have Sundays to ourselves while the two of you engage in 5-hour Bloody Mary brunches. Also, thanks for being pretty damn hot and sexy, too, and for saving us money on hiring fitness models for the pics in this book. ;-)

Thank you to our fitness models: Jill Coleman, Jillian Sarno Teta, Tara Ballard, and Jade Teta (who is anything but a fitness model, but we were desperate and he had to stand in). And thank you to our amazing photographer, Lisa Brewer.

A special thanks and big, huge hugs and kisses to our amazing agent, Celeste Fine. Thank you for being a dream keeper for so many, including us. There is no way to describe you other than magical! Thank you for all you have done and all you do, making this book and so many other books possible.

Thank you to our writer, Stephanie Krikorian, who had to put up with Jade's stress. Anyone who can make sense of his combination of PhD lingo and third-grade spelling deserves a medal.

To Jennifer Levesque, Jess Fromm, and the entire team at Rodale: Thank you for getting what this book was about from the start. We could not have found a better home for the book. Thank you for your amazing attention to detail and all you did in making this book come to life.

Gary Leake: Love you, man. Thanks for all you do. You are our rock. Without you, Keoni would not even know how to log on to the Internet, and Jade would have no place to vent all his stupid ideas.

Dan Coleman: You are the space maker, man. There need to be way more people like you in this world. Thanks for bringing the happy wherever you go without even trying.

Wilkey: Without you, Keoni would likely run away and never come back.

Dr. Ray Hinish: You, our friend, are one of the kindest, most selfless people we have ever met. In a world where ego and status often dominate, it is rare to find someone like you who just loves to see people succeed. Thanks for being in our corner. We feel stronger because of it.

Kimo Teta, we love the hell out of you, big brother. Thanks for always having our backs.

Jodi Teta: Love you, sis. Thanks for always putting up with us, for feeding us, and for being there no matter what. We hope you know we will always have your back like you have ours.

Lincoln Bryden: Thanks for putting up with Jade, Gary, and the rest of the ME team and their nonsense. We consider you family, man. Thanks for all you do every day spreading the ME message.

Esther Blum: How could we not forever just love the hell out of you? Thank you for who you are in the world. We so love you and admire who you are.

To the Metabolic Effect coaches: Erika Nall, Alan Bickmer, Joanne Morse, Christine Biswabic, Sara Lynn Johnson Baker. Thank you for all the work you do in the trenches every single day guiding thousands through our online programs. You are the lifeblood of Metabolic Effect, and your passion and knowledge inspire us every day.

To John Stevens: Love you bro. Thanks for all your work.

To all the health, fitness, weight-loss, and Internet marketing professionals in the trenches every single day, sharing your knowledge and passion with the world: Thank you for doing this work. There are many of you. Some we know and some we don't, but we would like to acknowledge those who we feel have especially enhanced our growth personally as professionals and whose information has had direct or indirect influence on this work: Jonny Bowden, Jen Sinkler, Neghar Fonooni, Brad Davidson, Daniel and Tana Amen, Liz Dialto, Sean Croxton, Christa Orecchio, Dave Dellanave, JJ Virgin, Jonathan Bailor, James Wedmore, Brad Pilon, Danny Gonzalez, John Berardi, Alwyn and Rachel Cosgrove, Ryan Halvorson, Molly Galbraith, Brooke Kalanick, Peter Hass, John Romaniello, Tom Venuto, Alan Aragon, Jen Comas Keck, Chris and Dani Shugart, Dr. David Katz, Dan Duchaine, Stephen Guyenet, Bill Phillips, Jeff Bland, Armand Morin, Brendon Burchard, Adam Bornstein, Amy Porterfield, Marc Stockman, Jeff Radich, Ramona Russell, and Ann Marie Gardner.

Notes and Sources

Introduction

Miller. "How Effective Are Traditional Dietary and Exercise Interventions for Weight Loss?" *Medicine and Science in Sports and Exercise* 31, no. 8 (Aug. 1999): 1129–34. ncbi.nlm.nih.gov /pubmed/10449014.

Mann, Tomiyama, Westling, Lew, Samuels, and Chatman. "Medicare's Search for Effective Obesity Treatments; Diets Are Not the Answer." *American Psychologist* 62, no. 3 (Apr. 2007): 220–33. ncbi.nlm.nih.gov/pubmed/17469900.

Chapter 1

Soenen, Martens, Hochstenbach-Waelen, Lemmens, and Westerterp-Plantenga. "Normal Protein Intake Is Required for Body Weight Loss and Weight Maintenance, and Elevated Protein Intake for Additional Preservation of Resting Energy Expenditure and Fat Free Mass." *Journal of Nutrition* 143, no. 5 (May 2013): 591–6. doi: 10.3945/jn.112.167593. ncbi.nlm.nih.gov/pubmed/23446962.

Tremblay, Royer, Chaput, and Doucet. "Adaptive Thermogenesis Can Make a Difference in the Ability of Obese Individuals to Lose Body Weight." *International Journal of Obesity* 37 (2013): 759–64.

Rosenbaum, Hirsch, Gallagher, and Leibel. "Long-Term Persistence of Adaptive Thermogenesis in Subjects Who Have Maintained a Reduced Body Weight." *American Society for Clinical Nutrition* 88, no. 4 (Oct. 2008): 906–12. ajcn.nutrition.org/content/88/4/906.long.

Miller and Parsonage. "Resistance to Slimming Adaptation or Illusion?" *Lancet* 305, no. 7910 (Apr. 1975): 773–5. doi:10.1016/S0140-6736(75)92437-X.

Hansen, Dendale, Berger, van Loon, and Meeusen. "The Effects of Exercise Training on Fat-Mass Loss in Obese Patients During Energy Intake Restriction." *Sports Medicine* 37, no. 1 (Jan. 2007): 31–46.

Bryner, Ullrich, Sauers, Donley, Hornsby, Kolar, and Yeater. "Effects of Resistance vs. Aerobic Training Combined with an 800 Calorie Liquid Diet on Lean Body Mass and Resting Metabolic Rate." *Journal of the American College of Nutrition* 18, no. 2 (Apr. 1999): 115–21.

Chapter 2

Teta and Teta. *The Metabolic Effect Diet: Eat More, Work Out Less, and Actually Lose Weight While You Rest.* New York: HarperCollins, 2010.

Chapter 5

Teta. "How to Stop Food Cravings: Understanding Trigger and Buffer Foods." MetabolicEffect.com, March 22, 2012. metaboliceffect.com/how-to-stop-food-cravings.

Hoyt, Hickey, and Cordain. "Dissociation of the Glycaemic and Insulinaemic Responses to Whole and Skimmed Milk." *British Journal of Nutrition* 93, no. 2 (Feb. 2005): 175–7.

Akcay and Akcay. "The Presence of the Antigliadin Antibodies in Autoimmune Thyroid Diseases." *Hepatogastroenterology* 50, Suppl. 2 (Dec. 2003): CCLXXIX–CCLXXX.

Chapter 6

Teta, Bessinger, and Bowden. *Natural Solutions for Digestive Health.* New York: Sterling, 2014.

Teta and Teta. "The Science Behind Rest Based Training (RBT)." metraineracademy.com/the-science-behind-rest-based-training-rbt.

Chapter 7

La Fleur, van Rozen, Luijenkijk, Groenwewg, and Adan. "A Free-Choice High-Fat High-Sugar Diet Induces Changes in Arcuate Neuropeptide Expression that Support Hyperphagia." *International Journal of Obesity* 34, no. 3 (Mar. 2010): 537–46. doi: 10.1038/ijo.2009.257.

Rising, Alger, Boyce, Seagle, Ferraro, Fontvieille, and Ravussin. "Food Intake Measured by an Automated Food-Selection System: Relationship to Energy Expenditure." *American Journal of Clinical Nutrition* 55 (Feb. 1992): 343–9.

Kadooka, Sato, Imaizumi, Ogawa, Ikuyama, Akai, Okano, Kagoshima, and Tsuchida. "Regulation of Abdominal Adiposity by Probiotics (*Lactobacillus gasseri* SBT2055) in Adults with Obese Tendencies in a Randomized Controlled Trial." *European Journal of Clinical Nutrition* 64, no. 6 (Jun. 2010): 636–43. doi: 10.1038/ejcn.2010.19.

Kurzweil and Grossman. *Transcend: Nine Steps to Living Well Forever.* New York: Rodale Books, 2010.

Chapter 8

Teta. "Ten Healthiest Fat Loss Foods." MetabolicEffect.com, April 11, 2012. metaboliceffect.com/10-healthiest-fat-loss-foods.

Kuo, Czarnecka, Kitlinska, Tilan, Kvetnansky, and Zukowska. "Chronic Stress, Combined with a High-Fat/High-Sugar Diet, Shifts Sympathetic Signaling toward Neuropeptide Y and Leads to Obesity and the Metabolic Syndrome." *Annals of the New York Academy of Sciences* 1148 (Dec. 2008): 232–7. doi: 10.1196/annals.1410.035.

Tomiyama, Mann, Vinas, Hunger, DeJager, and Taylor. "Low Calorie Dieting Increases Cortisol." *Psychosomatic Medicine* 72, no. 4 (May 2010): 357–64. doi: 10.1097/PSY.0b013e3181d9523c.

Foster, Wyatt, Hill, Makris, Rosenbaum, Brill, Stein, Mohammed, Miller, Rader, Zemel, Wadden, Tenhave, Newcomb, and Klein. "Weight and Metabolic Outcomes After 2 Years on a Low-Carbohydrate Versus Low-Fat Diet: A Randomized Trial." *Annals of Internal Medicine* 153, no. 3 (Aug. 2010): 147–57. doi:10.7326/0003-4819-153-3-201008030-00005.

Chapter 9

Kirchengast and Huber. "Body Composition Characteristics and Body Fat Distribution in Lean Women with Polycystic Ovary Syndrome." *Human Reproduction* 16, no. 6 (2001): 1255–60. doi: 10.1093/humrep/16.6.1255.

Wei, Zhao, Wang, Sui, Liang, Deng, Ma, Zhang, Zhang, and Guan. "A Clinical Study on the Short-Term Effect of Berberine in Comparison to Metformin on the Metabolic Characteristics of Women with Polycystic Ovary Syndrome." *European Journal of Endocrinology* 166, no. 1 (Jan. 2012): 99–105. doi: 10.1530/EJE-11-0616.

Xu, Ku, Tie, Yao, Jiang, Ma, and Li. "Curcumin Reverses the Effects of Chronic Stress on Behavior, the HPA Axis, BDNF Expression and Phosphorylation of CREB." *Brain Research* 1122, no. 1 (Nov. 2006): 56–64.

Hu, Lin, Lian, Zhou, Guo, Zhou, Chu, and Ge. "Curcumin as a Potent and Selective Inhibitor or 11ß-Hydroxysteroid Dehydrogenase 1: Improving Lipid Profiles in High-Fat-Diet-Treated Rats." *PLoS One* 8, no. 3 (2013). doi: 10.1371/journal.pone.0049976.

Tiwari-Pandey and Ram Sairam. "Modulation of Ovarian Structure and Abdominal Obesity in Curcumin- and Flutamide-Treated Aging FSH-R Haploinsufficient Mice." *Reproductive Sciences* 16, no. 6 (Jun. 2009): 539–50. doi: 10.1177/1933719109332822.

Cosar, Uçok, Akgün, Köken, Sahin, Arioz, and Bas. "Body Fat Composition and Distribution in Women with Polycystic Ovary Syndrome." *Gynecological Endocrinology* 24, no. 8 (Aug. 2008): 428–32. doi: 10.1080/09513590802234253.

Casazza, Jacobs, Suh, Iller, Horning, and Brooks. "Menstrual Cycle Phase and Oral Contraceptive Effects on Triglyceride Mobilization During Exercise." *Journal of Applied Physiology* 97 (July 2004): 302–9. doi: 10.1152/japplphysiol.00050.2004.

Davidsen, Vistisen, and Astrup. "Impact of the Menstrual Cycle on Determinants of Energy Balance: A Putative Role in Weight Loss Attempts." *International Journal of Obesity* 31, no. 12 (Dec. 2007): 1777–85.

D'Eon and Braun. "The Roles of Estrogen and Progesterone in Regulating Carbohydrate and Fat Utilization at Rest and During Exercise." *Journal of Women's Health and Gender-Based Medicine* 11, no. 3 (2002): 225–37.

Nakamura, Aizawa, Imai, Kono, and Mesaki. "Hormonal Responses to Resistance Exercise During Different Menstrual Cycle States." *Medicine and Science in Sports and Exercise* 43, no. 6 (Jun. 2011): 967–73. doi: 10.1249/MSS.0b013e3182019774.

Oosthuyse and Bosch. "The Effect of the Menstrual Cycle on Exercise Metabolism." *Sports Medicine* 40, no. 3 (Mar. 2010): 207–27. doi: 10.2165/11317090-000000000-00000.

Matsuo, Saitoh, and Suzuki. "Effects of the Menstrual Cycle on Excess Postexercise Oxygen Consumption in Healthy Young Women." *Metabolism* 48, no. 3 (Mar. 1999): 275–7.

Davis, Wood, Andrews, Elkind, and Davis. "Concurrent Training Enhances Athletes' Strength, Muscle Endurance, and Other Measures." *Journal of Strength and Conditioning Research* 22, no. 5 (Sep. 2008): 1487–502. doi: 10.1519/JSC.0b013e3181739f08.

Index

Boldface page references indicate illustrations and photographs. <u>Underscored</u> references indicate boxed text.

for new routine, 27, 30
  protein, 205
  quantifying, 45
  steps to fix, 28–30
    balance the brain, 30
    hack the habit, 28–30
    pay attention, 28
Curcumin, 200

D

Dairy products, 64–65, 77–78, 102, 172
Decline pushup, 91
Depression, 148–49
Diet
  biases, 43
  carb-to-protein-to-fat ratio in, 75
  creating individual, 41–54
    adjustments to get HEC in check, 50–51, 51
    AIM process, 51–54
    as diet detective, 42–43
    keeping HEC in check, 44–47, 100–103
    measuring results, 47–49, **49**
    practicing to achieve mastery, 42
    preconceived notions, putting aside, 43
    structured flexibility, 44, 45
    when you are not burning fat, 49–51, 51
  cycling, 17, 31, 95–96, 127, 140
  digestive restoration, 150–53
  perfect, 41–42
  plant-based, 145
  for targeting stubborn fat
    back-of-the-arm fat, 201
    belly blast protocol, 200
    love handles, 207
    lower-body blast protocol, 195
    male belly fat, 205
Diet detective, 41–54
  exercise recovery, 153–54
  maintenance phase approaches, 133–34
  sleep, 154–55
  wine and alcohol, 61
Dieting
  compensatory effects of, 14–15
  fad diets, 2
  failure, 14, 42
  focusing on calories, 29
  stress of, 3, 19
  trap, 42–43, 53, 134, 169
  willpower drain of, 216, 218
Digestion
  as biofeedback clue, 112–13, 149
  Digestive Restorative Program, 150–53
  protein, 68
Digestive enzyme products, 68, 151
Digestive enzymes, dilution of, 64
Dining out on 4-2-2 eating plan, 105

Dinner plate, 3-2-1, 61, **61**
Dopamine, 21, 26, 30, 112, 197

E

Eating
  after workouts, 114–15, 132, 179, 181
  behavioral, 63, 63
  carbohydrate timing strategies, 179–81
  4-2-2 eating plan, 96, **96**, 98–115
  frequency, 182
  thermogenic effect of, 168
  3-2-1 eating plan, 60–61, **61**, 63–81
  too little, 108–9
Eat Less, Exercise Less (ELEL) approach/phase
  alternating with EMEM approach, 96, 127
  belly fat targeted by, 38, 38–39
  biochemical hunger control during, 23–24
  cycling the diet, 17, 96, 127
  fasting overnight to begin, 60
  HGH and testosterone elevation with, 18
  in maintenance phase, 129, 131, 140–42, **141**
  menstrual cycle and, 22
  overview, 59–62
  3-2-1 eating plan, 60–61, **61**, 63–81
    buffer foods, 79–80
    calorie deficit, untraditional, 80–81
    crushing cravings, 72–76
    5-4-1 approach for cravings, 66
    overview, 60–61, **61**
    protein meals, 66–67
    protein ratio calculator, 74–75
    protein shakes, 63–65
    recipes, 69–72
    spices, 68–69
    3-2-1 dinner plate, 61, **61**
    trigger foods, 76–79
  3-2-1 exercise plan, 61, 81–92
    equipment, 86
    exercise obsessed, 92
    moving *versus* exercise, 81–82
    overview, 61
    rest and recovery activities, 61–62, 85–86
    smart exercise, 83–84
    walking, 61–62, 82, 84, 92
    weight training, 61–62, 86–91, 87, **88–91**
    workout, 86, 87
  3-2-1 sample week, 62
Eat Less, Exercise More approach, 140, **141**
  avoiding, 8, 13, 17, 24
  effects of
    energy level decrease, 24
    hormonal imbalance, 31
    metabolic adjustments, 3–4
    skinny fat body type, 10
  focusing on calories, 29
Eat More, Exercise Less approach, 140, **141**

love handles, 206–8
male belly fat, <u>38</u>, 205–6
male chest fat, 208–9
subcutaneous fat, 36–37, 198, 206–7
visceral fat, 36–37, 198
receptors in fat tissue, 34–37
science of, 33–36
stubborn fat
alpha- and beta-adrenergic receptors and,
34–35, 37
blood flow to, 34–35, 37
description of, 36–37
diet adjustment for burning, 50
effectiveness in burning, monitoring,
47–48
fat release from, 34–35
female *versus* male, **36**, 37, <u>38</u>
location of, **36**, 36–37, 191–210
physiology of, 33–39
storage, estrogen and, 22, 35
targeting, 37–39, <u>38</u>, 191–210
Fat(s) (dietary fat)
adding to get HEC in check, 46, 53, <u>103</u>, 172
carb-to-protein-to-fat ratio in diet, <u>75</u>
combined with starch, sugar, or salt, 78, 146,
173–76
cutting back in diet, 50–51, <u>51</u>, <u>103</u>
fat-gain formula, 175–76
in fat-loss-food cheat sheet, <u>100</u>
tips for, 104
vegetable fat, 172
Fat burning
diet modifying when you are not burning fat,
49–51, <u>51</u>
hormone-sensitive lipase and, 33–35
hormones involved, 18–19, 34–35
adrenaline, 18, 21, 34–35
cortisol, 18, 20–21
estrogen, 22
GLP (glucagon-like peptide), 20
human growth hormone, 18, 205
thyroid hormone, 19
with metabolic conditioning, 117–20
myth of simultaneous muscle building, <u>5</u>, <u>29</u>
process of, <u>34</u>
stubborn fat, 47–48, 50
Fat gain, stress and, 174–77
Fat-gain formula, 175–76
Fat loss
adrenergic receptors and, 34–35
diet modifying when you are not burning fat,
49–51, <u>51</u>
muscle loss *versus,* 7
resistance training *versus* aerobic exercise, 7
Fat-loss foods, 104–5, 168–74
cheat sheet, <u>100–103</u>
green foods, <u>170</u>, 171

red foods, <u>170</u>, 172–74
yellow foods, <u>170</u>, 171–72
Fat storage
alcohol and, <u>61</u>
body's assessment of stores, <u>60</u>
body's defense of fat stores, 3
food effects on, <u>170</u>
hormones involved, 19–22, 34–35
cortisol, 21
estrogen, 22
GIP (glucose-dependent insulinotropic
peptide), 20
insulin, 19–20, 34–35, <u>38</u>
NPY (neuropeptide Y), 21
progesterone, 22
lipoprotein lipase and, 33–34
location of, **36**, 36–37
Feeding the lean approach, 17, 22–24, 31,
<u>38</u>. *See also* Eat More, Exercise More
(EMEM) approach/phase
Fiber
adding to get HEC in check, 46, 53, 72
adding to protein shake, <u>107</u>
hunger control with, <u>24</u>, 72
sources
carbohydrate foods, 11–12
fat-loss foods, 169
nonstarchy vegetables, 205
starchy foods, 98
supplement, 72
starch-to-fiber ratio, 173
toxin binding by, 9, 13
Fitbit, 82
5-alpha reductase, 29
5-4-1 approach for cravings, <u>66</u>
5-hydroxytryptophan, 30
Flavor in foods, 68–69, 78
Flexibility, structured, 6, 44, 45, <u>74</u>
Food addiction, 143–46, 174
Foods
best carb-based foods, 12
buffer, 79–80
combinations, 78, 146, 173–76
fat-loss, <u>100–103</u>, 104–5, 168–74
flavor, 68–69, 78
4-2-2 eating plan, 96, **96**, 98–115
highly palatable, 78, 142–46
immune reactions to, 77–78, <u>102</u>,
149–53, 178–79
negative-calorie, 73
nutrient dense, 12
preconceived notions, putting aside, 43
3-2-1 eating plan, 60–61, **61**, 63–81
trigger, 76–79
water content, 11–12, <u>24</u>, 73, 169,
173
Food sensitivities/allergies, <u>60</u>, 149–53

4-2-2 protocol
   4-2-2 eating plan, 96, **96**, 98–115
   4-2-2 exercise plan, 97, 115–26
   4-2-2 sample week, 97–98
Fruits
   high water *versus* low water *versus* high
      sugar, <u>100</u>
   low-sugar, 177
   as trigger foods, 78

G

GABA (gamma-aminobutyric acid), 21, 30, 74,
   112, <u>155</u>
Garlic, 69
Gas, <u>68</u>, 72, 112, 149
Gastric bypass surgery, 20
Ghrelin, 8, 19, 25, <u>93</u>, <u>189</u>
Ginger, 68, 111
GIP (glucose-dependent insulinotropic
   peptide), 20
Giving, 216–17
GLP (glucagon-like peptide), 20, 73
Glucose, fasting, <u>160</u>
Glutamate, 30
Glutamine, 152
Gluten, 77–78, 179
Glycation, <u>156–57</u>, <u>161</u>
Glycogen depletion, 195, <u>196</u>
Grains, 173, **173**, 179
Gratitude, 217
Green coffee extract, 200
Green tea extract, <u>8</u>, 192–93, <u>195</u>, 195–96, 207

H

Habit loop, 27, <u>63</u>
Habits
   behavioral hunger and, 25
   breaking, 27–28, <u>63</u>
   cravings and, 27–30
Halo effect, 82–83
Heart rate, waking, 188
Heart rate recovery, 188
Heart rate variability, 188–89
Heavy bench press, 91
HEC (hunger, energy, and cravings). *See also*
   Cravings; Energy; Hunger
   in AIM process, 51–54
   carbohydrates and, 11, 104
   cheat sheet, <u>24</u>
   exercise impact on, 83–84
   fluctuations in, 44–45
   getting/keeping in check, 6–7, 44–47
      diet adjustments to balance, 50–51, <u>51</u>,
         <u>100–103</u>
      in ELEL phase, 72–76

      in EMEM phase, <u>108</u>, 108–9, 113–14
      fat-loss foods, 168, <u>170</u>
      in maintenance phase, 142–46, <u>143</u>
      steps to take, 45–47
   indicator of hormone balance, 18, 26, <u>29</u>, 44
   quantifying, 45
   reproductive hormone influence on, 21–22
   trigger foods, 76–79
Hemoglobin A1c, <u>160–61</u>
HGH, 18, 118, <u>190</u>, 205
High-sensitivity C-reactive protein (hs-CRP),
   160–61
Homocysteine, <u>160–61</u>
Hormonal carbohydrate calculator, 11–12
Hormone replacement therapy, 204
Hormone resistance, 7, <u>93</u>
Hormones. *See also specific hormones*
   balance, 23, <u>29</u>
      causes of changes in, 147–48
      for craving control, 30
      HEC as indicator of, 18, 26, <u>29</u>, 44
   fat-burning, 18–19
   fat storage and release, effects on, 34–36
   Goldilocks zone for levels of, <u>93</u>
   HEC, influence on, 6–7, 18
   how they work, 23
   hunger, 19–20, 23–26
   incretins, 20
   love handles and, 207
   metabolic myths concerning, <u>29</u>
   reproductive, 21–22, 35–36
   stress, 20–21
Hormone-sensitive lipase, 33–37
Hourglass body shape, 22, <u>47</u>, 47–48, **49**, <u>158</u>
hs-CRP, <u>160–61</u>
Human growth hormone (HGH), 18, 118, <u>190</u>,
   205
Hunger. *See also* HEC (hunger, energy, and
   cravings)
   behavioral, 23–25, <u>24</u>, <u>60</u>, <u>64</u>, 112
   biochemical, 23, 25
   difference from cravings, 25–26, 112, <u>113</u>
   exercises decreasing, 84
   exercises increasing, 83–84
   fasting and, 183–84, <u>186</u>, 187
   Goldilocks zone, <u>93</u>
   high-fat, high-sugar foods and, 176
   hormones involved, 19–20, <u>24</u>, 25
      ghrelin, 8, 19, 25
      GIP (glucose-dependent insulinotropic
         peptide), 20
      GLP (glucagon-like peptide), 20, 73
      insulin, 8, 19, <u>24</u>, <u>93</u>
      leptin, 8, 19, <u>24</u>, <u>93</u>
      NPY (neuropeptide Y), 21, 175–77
   inability to control as sign of metabolic
      damage, <u>8</u>